Erotic Dreams

Erotic Dreams

The Secret to Understanding Women's Hidden Passions

GILLIAN HOLLOWAY, PH.D.

A PERIGEE BOOK

A PERIGEE BOOK
Published by the Penguin Group
Penguin Group (USA) Inc.
375 Hudson Street, New York, New York 10014, USA
Penguin Group (Canada), 90 Eglinton Avenue East, Suite 700, Toronto, Ontario M4P 2Y3, Canada
(a division of Pearson Penguin Canada Inc.)
Penguin Books Ltd., 80 Strand, London WC2R 0RL, England
Penguin Group Ireland, 25 St. Stephen's Green, Dublin 2, Ireland (a division of Penguin Books Ltd.)
Penguin Group (Australia), 250 Camberwell Road, Camberwell, Victoria 3124, Australia
(a division of Pearson Australia Group Pty. Ltd.)
Penguin Books India Pvt. Ltd., 11 Community Centre, Panchsheel Park, New Delhi—110 017, India
Penguin Group (NZ), Cnr. Airborne and Rosedale Roads, Albany, Auckland 1310, New Zealand
(a division of Pearson New Zealand Ltd.)
Penguin Books (South Africa) (Pty.) Ltd., 24 Sturdee Avenue, Rosebank, Johannesburg 2196,
South Africa

Penguin Books Ltd., Registered Offices: 80 Strand, London WC2R 0RL, England

While the author has made every effort to provide accurate telephone numbers and Internet addresses at the time of publication, neither the publisher nor the author assumes any responsibility for errors, or for changes that occur after publication. Further, publisher does not have any control over and does not assume any responsibility for author or third-party websites or their content.

First edition: August 2006

Library of Congress Cataloging-in-Publication Data

Holloway, Gillian.
  Erotic dreams : the secret to understanding women's hidden passions / Gillian Holloway.
  p. cm.
  ISBN 0-399-53262-5
1. Sex in dreams. 2. Sex symbolism. 3. Women's dreams. I. Title.
  BF1099.S4H65 2006
  154.6'32—dc22
                                        2006014142

PRINTED IN THE UNITED STATES OF AMERICA

10 9 8 7 6 5 4 3 2 1

CONTENTS

PART 4

The Mystical Side

PART 5

Accepting Your Power and Passion

Introduction

Look! No Hands

I had a dream a year or so ago in which I was attending a going-away party. There was a man, a middle-aged doctor who was going away to practice in Europe. Though I didn't know him, I was a friend of the group of women who were giving him a send-off. I noticed he was a double amputee, and that he had the old-fashioned prosthetic hands that were like hooks. He sat smiling with a gift on his lap while the women talked and laughed around him, obviously very fond of him. I was touched; he had finished medical school late in life, and with something of a handicap, but he seemed either unaware of this or uninterested in it. He was focused on his mission.

In the dream I saw him again, running into him in a shopping area. I ran up to him and threw my arms around him, realizing too late that he didn't seem to recognize me. Nevertheless he embraced me. As I pulled back I reminded him that we had met at the party, and he seemed gently amused that I was so flustered. I just felt a huge affection for him.

In the next scene of the dream, I was visiting this doctor in Italy, where he had set his practice. As we talked, there was a kind of sexual electricity that was moving around the room. We were discussing his medical practice, but I was having trouble listening to what he was saying. Finally I bolted over to him, jumped in his lap, and we kissed. I had the shaky sex-is-inevitable feeling, and with a certain amount of fumbling we were soon on the floor. Somehow, I was able to read his mind, and I knew it had been a long time for him, since before the accident that took his hands. It had been a long time for me, too, and I had a moment's concern that I might not be up to speed, sexually. But then I caught him worrying about his disfigurement, and I wanted him to know I *so* didn't care about that; I could eat him like a mint. At the same time I realized I'd have to put him on his back and be a little proactive, because it didn't look like he could balance on his elbows or be on top. The sensation of being close to him was both emotionally and sexually delicious, and every touch was tender and urgent. Afterward, I curled up with him like a cat who is making a nest, feeling very much at home.

When I awoke from this dream, I knew it was important, not only because it was unusual but also because of the strong feelings involved. If this were simply a fantasy for the release of tension, why would my mind create a middle-aged balding man without hands? Why did I love him, as well as want to have sex with him? I took the dream to my personal group of dream friends and shared it during one of our regular meetings. One of the members, Tracy, said, "I don't know what this means, but I think you should write more, and I think you should write about sex."

She was more accurate than she realized. While I am regularly interviewed about women's sexual dreams, for some reason it had not occurred to me until that moment to do a book on them. It was then, in that dream meeting, and because of that dream, that this project was born. I think that the aging doctor who had lost his hands represents a part of me that feels past her prime, who has for too long postponed the soul-nourishing work of writing. (This is what took the hands away, procrastination.)

Years earlier I had a dream about a friend of mine who is a writer, and in this dream she, too, had lost her hands. This was yet another memo from my subconscious that said, "The writer has lost her action." While this sounds creepy, women often dream of injuries to the hands and even of amputated hands and fingers. It's more common than you would imagine. In the broadest sense, the theme of hand loss or injury seems associated with loss of some activity, some autonomy or authority or identity. It is loss of some aspect of self, related to independence and being in the world.

In this "no-hands" dream, we see the superficial trappings of the encapsulated setting that permits sexuality to emerge instead of being distracted or neglected. I visit the doctor in Italy (land of passion and romance, perhaps?). He has been living a neutered, purposeful life because of being unsure whether anyone would want him, which makes my own awkwardness no big deal.

Intrapsychically this dream shows that what I really want, what turns me on most, is a sense of purpose, contributing, and moving forward whether you have some scars or all your parts or whatever. In order to have this, the dream hints, I have to be more proactive than usual. I have to essentially jump on this thing, consummate the passion, and connect with what I love. The heartfelt quality of this dream and the *oomph* of the passion let me know that even if the interpretation was a little hazy or general, I had to move toward both writing and passion.

Even women who don't usually remember dreams tend to recall erotic dreams. Whether the dream entailed the best sex of your life, an orgasmic tango, or the electric shock of a first kiss, you may ponder it for some time.

Some erotic dreams come in clusters, so that the same dream figure guest stars in a series of fantasy encounters or stalking nightmares. When the themes are negative, we worry the dreams are warnings of trouble ahead. If the dreams are great, we wonder if a new lover is coming down the pike, or if the satisfying scenes in the dream represent factors that would heat up real-life intimacy.

What's In It for You

Erotic dreams and fantasies are so intriguing, sexy, and fun that they do have entertainment value. You might get a laugh from a friend by sharing your dream of a sexy circus act, or take time to listen to her dream of straddling the blowhole of a whale. But our dreams and fantasies are more than curiosities: They are illustrations of feelings. By taking a look at this collection of dreams and fantasies, you may see how your own compare and what themes modern women share.

To some extent we are all scattering our fire these days: more determined than ever to have what we want, but sometimes distracted by the speed at which we fly and the array of choices that surround us. We know we can have almost anything, yet sometimes feel haunted by the fear that we are destined to have everything except the thing we want most.

Start a Dream Journal

One of the best ways to fulfill your passions is to understand your dreams. Find a way, right now, to begin to record your dreams; whether you recall epic sagas or fleeting images is unimportant. Type dreams into your computer, record them vocally, or jot them into a notebook of some kind. Expect and insist on remembering one dream a week at a minimum. Keep a means of recording dreams handy by your bedside, the less fuss involved, the better. Doing the work of recording your dreams, then reviewing their meaning, will, in itself, impact your dreaming patterns. The scenes will be more vivid, the dream stories more cohesive like movies, and your memory will become much stronger. Best of all, by thoughtfully reviewing your dreams for meaning, you'll find that your dreams become sensitive to your suggestions, and you will get *answers*.

Don't worry about interpreting a dream the moment you have it. Record it and then return to it later. You'll find that the distance of a little time will make the meaning much easier to identify. Instead of worry or blame, you'll be able to pick out the gem of insight the dream has for you. If you are interested in joining or starting a dream-sharing group, I'll provide directions on how to find one or get one started in the final chapter of the book.

Differences Between Dreams and Fantasies

Fantasy Qualities

Fantasies are usually sensation amplifiers: taking the thread of a stimulating idea or memory and exaggerating it through extreme circumstance or multiplication to create a portable "orgasmatron" in your mind. While fantasies are usually about something fun and stimulating, they are often not something we literally want to have happen or to play out on the same scale. The revved-up engines of our fantasies are meant to take us over the edge when we're alone, or trying (presto-sexo) to snap out of fatigue and into passion. To review a fantasy for possible real-life implications, we need to ask what element is being blown out of proportion and whether is makes any kind of sense to strike that chord in real life.

Dream Qualities

Erotic dreams tend to be more abstract than fantasies and to incorporate more unexpected events. While the involuntary, symbolic quality of dreams makes them tougher to understand and remember, they are also loaded with potential gold that has real-world value for the dreamer.

Imagine that you could take a core sample from the essence of your being that would incorporate your history, your personality, your larger potentials, your sexual appetite, and your overall life goals. The material of our dreams is comprised of that mix, thrown against a blank canvas over and over, forming by the weight of its elements into plots and episodes that mirror current tensions, fantasies, and frustrations.

Erotic dreams are more than imaginary blips on the night-time screen, they are guts-and-blood artwork of the soul, not always revealing fantasy sex, but always exploring real passion. You may dream of sex with a scientist, not because you want to "do" one, but because you want to *be* one. By watching how these themes play out, we can perhaps discover the essence behind the forms in our dreams. By examining what goes wrong in our dreams, we can position ourselves with greater balance and awareness in the real world to avoid disappointment or sabotage.

The Four Payoffs of Erotic Dreams

Sexual Insight: Improving Sex

Some sexy dreams are like dessert with no calories. Yummy adventures with no consequences often parallel our sexual fantasies. These dreams show us what is fun and why. The imaginary partners or ideal settings hint at qualities that combine risk with safety, privacy with the envy of strangers who may pass by. While these dreams infuse us with pleasure, they also sometimes reveal qualities that can make our connections deeper and more satisfying.

Self-Understanding: Improving Life

Many erotic dreams are "intrapsychic" dramas. Some of our best dream lovers symbolize potentials in ourselves that are constructed from our deepest passions. That doctor in the Everglades may not be your fantasy guy; it is equally possible he is a part of *you* that seems like too much of a long shot to express in real life. As we adapt to life and play the cards we're dealt, we also hedge our bets and underestimate ourselves. But our talents and passions are like dormant volcanoes sending up plumes of smoke in our dreams. The erotic meltdowns in these dreams are sometimes more haunting than real sex, because we have had a taste of consummating a passion that has burned for a lifetime.

Relationship Views: Improving Connections

Though deciphering and benefiting from our dreams has long been controversial (and taboo), many researchers now agree that dreams tend to focus on our current situations and can solve problems. While dreams don't always lay out solutions in point-blank style, they are *drawn* to our unfinished business, recurring dilemmas, or blocks with seemingly endless persistence. Our erotic dreams often straddle the twin points of desire and frustration, creating stories about what is out of whack and how to fix it.

Destiny Distortions: Course Corrections

Finally, erotic dreams are so mingled with all of our passions that there is frequently a bleed-through effect. We begin to have dreams of stunning passion at times when the window is open for us to make a change or explore an avenue so potent, so compelling, it appears *meant to be*.

This doesn't mean we automatically become rich or famous for a heretofore unrecognized talent, but it does mean that life can be transformed from black-and-white to Technicolor in the degree of aliveness we feel at expressing ourselves in the real world. When we don't express something we are meant to express, there is a diminution of vitality that pervades our feelings and perspectives. It is as if we have a kink in the hose, or a distortion in our destiny, and although everything is "right," something feels wrong.

Dreams are one of the best ways to find out what this subjective mystery is all about. Our passionate stories are drenched with the serum of what will make our lives flow and our spirits unfold. This is when each sexual stroke in a dream is like a stroke of lightning; when we connect, even in imagination, with our unlived possibilities, it is truly amazing.

The Material, Conception, and Birth of This Book

I live and work in the world of the imagination, teaching courses on dreamwork, intuition, and storytelling at Marylhurst University in the Pacific Northwest. An early interest in dreams led me to study with Gayle Delaney, PhD, and to explore the modern themes and symbols that many of us have in common in our dreams. For the past ten years, the Internet had enhanced the collection of dreams so that many researchers, myself included, are able to examine a great number of dreams and to see what situations, ages, and backgrounds may coincide with what types of dreams.

More women recall and share their dreams than do men, and perhaps women feel a greater intuition that the powerful feelings and stirring images of their dreams may be important to understand. Certainly there can be magic in the group sharing and exploration of dreams. Dreams take our everyday situations and turn them upside down; from that different angle we can often see how things fit together, or why some pattern is repeating in our lives.

For whatever reason, I have found myself involved in dream discussion groups. Without planning it, the all-female groups have at times afforded discussion of dreams that we might normally keep to ourselves because they were so personal, sexual, or shocking. In a kind of gentle wonder, we sometimes discover that one woman's dream holds solutions for all of us. You do not have to have had the same dream to be nourished by the underlying truth in another's story. It is as if some dreams not only hold potential gifts for the dreamer, but also may nourish and reassure others through some inexplicable alchemy of the imagination.

Most people who work with the analysis and interpretation of dreams will agree that the ultimate interpretation of any dream should come from the dreamer or at the very least from dialogue and mutual exploration with the dreamer.

As you read the descriptions of dreams in this book, maintain your authority, as the author of your dreams. Take what nourishes you from these stories, but don't attempt to try to force a parallel or analogy that doesn't ring true. It is exciting to theorize about why women have similar themes in erotic dreams, and to borrow from the discoveries of others to examine your own dreams. Use the experiences described here as a magnifying glass through which to take a closer look at your own themes.

Why Dreams and Fantasies

Women's dreams tend to have an edge of dissatisfaction and frustration to them, even when they are sexual fantasies. Researchers estimate that two-thirds of our dreams have elements of anxiety. Most women know that even our best sex dreams tend to take twists that change the tone or turn the hottest encounter into an *I Love Lucy* moment.

Most of the dreams in this book come from first-person explorations with the dreamers, some through correspondence. The fantasies come from women who responded to my requests of the last year for fantasies to see if these themes coincided with the dreams we have in common. The database of dreams is around twenty-eight thousand, while only a few thousand women were able to share fantasies. Some fantasies are included in part to give us a chance to see more wish-fulfillment themes without the intrusion of tensions that often short-circuit eroticism in our dreams.

The chapters in this book are clustered according to shared themes. Where possible, the chapters include discussion of a fantasy that echoes the same theme. We often dream of frustrations and interruptions, partners who evaporate or turn mean. But of course, we fantasize about what seems like fun. Because some chapters focus on nightmares or frustrations, those themes do not include parallel fantasies, but do explore the meaning and advantages the dreamers discovered through their understanding of the dreams.

Be Prepared

As you read this book, you may find your own dreams increasing erotic themes, particularly if you read just before bed. Your assignment, if you choose to accept it, is to record these themes and consider what, besides fun, they have to offer.

Each chapter concludes with an interactive exercise, called a dream key, that encourages you to take a self-test, apply principles to your own life, or explore themes and symbols. Not all of these keys will seem to apply to you, because some of the doors they unlock haven't shown up in your dreams. Just use these ideas as references and take what serves you. In some cases you may have dreams in the future that will be immediately meaningful instead of weird, because you will have given thought to the blueprints of your own symbolism.

PART ONE

Sizzle and Spark

CHAPTER ONE

Faceless Lovers

One of the most pervasive and enigmatic themes in erotic dreams deals with a lover who has no face. Sometimes his face is in the shadows and "accidentally" cannot be seen in the dream's action. Some women say that the lover is like a picture with the face airbrushed away, that there is a diffuse cloud where the face should be.

Still other women say that the entire lover is cloudy and indeterminate. The visceral connection is real, as are the sensations and excitement, but the person is impossible to identify. Perhaps the most provocative quality of these dreams is the experience of emotional intimacy and visceral chemistry dissociated from a personal identity of the partner. We may love and want and be thrilled by this being in the most personal ways, but we do not apparently need to know who he is in order to have these feelings.

Cloud Man

One woman reported she sometimes dreamed of a man who was vaporous like a cloud. A mist would gather in her room. As this mist grew close to her, the vapor grew denser and solidified into a lifelike form. In these dreams, she would always be surprised to find that the cloud had not only become a man, but that she and this cloud were having sex. The sensation of his solidity would intensify, as would her pleasure. Yet there was never the sense of having someone on top of her, or of being pressed down by the weight of a partner. The cloud remained almost weightless, while the sense of penetration, thrusting, and rhythmic rocking grew more real.

These dreams occurred during her single years, when she was often without a regular partner. When she had regular lovers and later a husband, the dream visits from this amorous cloud stopped. Perhaps on one level, her physical hunger for companionship caused her mind to coalesce this vapor into a form that could then satisfy her. But if her mind were "cooking up" a fantasy to satisfy her desire, why not something more substantial or resembling the Hollywood leading man of the day? She felt that perhaps during that time of her life, she had not the slightest idea of what she might want in a man, except to have sex. Her idea of what was desirable or right for her was completely hazy and unformed. In that sense, her fantasy came to her in dream form, very much as it was in her mind, completely mysterious, but bearing the gift of sexual pleasure.

Almost Zorro

A divorced woman said that for a few years she had periodic dreams of a man she would simply find wandering around her house. This man was not dangerous; in fact he was very attractive to her, although she could never quite see who he was. She had the dreams so often she came to recognize him in the hallway as "him" whenever she saw him. In these dreams she and the man would just stop and have sex wherever they encountered each other. In one dream she remembered lying back on the top of the stairs, while he knelt a few stairs below between her legs performing oral sex. In another encounter they were in her bedroom. He was behind her, caressing her, and she threw her head back in pleasure, but not before she barely glimpsed him in the mirror. In that moment she thought perhaps the shadow that always seemed to conceal his face was not a shadow but a *mask*. But she couldn't be sure.

During the year or two immediately after her divorce, this woman was still stinging from the experience. Although she ultimately wanted to remarry or have someone in her life, it took her a while to stop feeling cranky toward men. This phantom lover was a man of few words, no identity, and endless foreplay. There was nothing about him to resent or long for. No future, no past, no plans, and no disappointments. Perhaps the concealed face is sometimes a reprieve from all the parameters and requirements we, and society, place on our love lives. For this woman, "almost Zorro" was a fantasy treat that gave her positive experiences without risk, until she was ready to become close to someone again.

Faceless Groom

One woman has a recurring dream that she is finally getting the wedding she has wanted since childhood. Everything is perfect and detailed; her dress, the music, the beautiful church, and the friends and family who attend. She walks up the aisle with her father, approaches the groom, and stands beside him. She reaches out for his hand, and they stand together. He is wearing a stunning tuxedo and has a physique she finds attractive.

But at this point the dream becomes frustrating, for though she raises her eyes to look into his, she can't. This groom, who is otherwise perfect in every way, simply has no face.

On the most superficial level, this dream seems analogous to the sex dreams above. Only instead of creating sex without a commitment, this dream is about the wedding—the celebration and the promise involved. The dreamer knows in detail exactly what she wants; she just doesn't have a face to plug into the wedding pictures yet. But if this were the only trigger for this dream, why wouldn't her mind just put in the most handsome generic or celebrity face available? That would be more soothing than the disquiet she feels as she gazes lovingly in to Mr. No-face in his tuxedo. That's a bit disquieting, and even in the dream it is frustrating.

Perhaps there is a reason why it is important for her to keep this picture incomplete for a while. This wedding is beautiful, and there is no reason why she shouldn't want it and shouldn't have it. Yet intuitively her mind holds something back from the fantasy, and perhaps with good reason. The man's face represents the individual she will hope to marry, someone she has not found at the time of these dreams. While weddings are about planning, accessories, and catering, marriages are about people. Who she loves and is loved by could change everything she envisions and everything she wants. There is nothing wrong with her wonderful wedding dreams; they simply will not truly gel into life plans until she knows more about the partner that fate has in store.

Indigenous Ritual

When she became engaged, one woman had a lovely dream that she was part of an indigenous village somewhere. There was some kind of celebration going on, and she realized it was a wedding celebration. There was music and drumming; older people danced while children raced around laughing and squealing. There was a young man who came up to her and picked her up in his arms as if she weighed nothing at all. They laughed, and he then held her by her waist and spun around so that her legs flew out like a child. They ran, hand in hand, away from the others and into the forest, where they found a sheltered area and fell to the ground, pressing their bodies together.

This dream clearly reflected the woman's happiness at her engagement, and it also hinted that she had the feeling of coming home to herself in a personal sense. This village setting is like an original home, a place of connection and love.

The Ranch Hand

There are a number of photographs and posters that depict a lone cowboy on a horse, silhouetted against the sunset. It is impossible to see his face; there is just a strong man on horseback wearing a worn-looking cowboy hat. These posters are more effective because we cannot see this man's face. We can imagine him however we want him to be, or we can just enjoy the poetry the image suggests, uncomplicated by any hint of realism.

One woman reported a version of the faceless-lover dream involving a cowboy whose face was obscured by his hat. In the dream, she was outside curled up on a porch swing, when she heard the clump of boots climbing up wooden stairs. The swing creaked as a man sat down beside her and began running his hand along her shoulder and up behind her neck, lightly kneading the place where she often grew tense. Because of the twilight and the hat he wore, she could not see his face. She sighed as his warm hand relaxed her, and he leaned forward and put his lips on her throat. His arm slid around her waist, and he continued his explorations, only pausing to comment that she was the type of woman who would make a man wear himself out.

This gently sensual dream is full of promise and mystery. Not all dreams have action consistent with the setting and tone, but many do. In this sweet fantasy the man is slow-moving and admiring, waiting for her to incrementally relax before the dream becomes more sexual.

This scene also hints at some of the qualities the dreamer craves, more time, more relaxation, admiration, and recognition. She is on a porch swing, hardly a place of raucous orgies.

Porch swings are for slow twilights and easygoing times. The setting, the fantasy lover, and the action are all slow-moving and allow her time to recover from her tensions before she begins to notice sexual feelings brewing.

Dream Key #1

What Qualities Do You Value Most?

Once we take away the superficial dazzle of an alluring face, we are to some extent left with the qualities of behavior and the emotional flavor of a fantasy lover. If you have fallen for someone who looked good but behaved badly, you already know there is something important about understanding what qualities you appreciate and need in a partner. Answer the questions below, rating each trait with the higher numbers indicating highest importance. When you are done, make yourself a little list of the things that are most important to you. If there is something not listed below that is vital to you, add it to the list.

Sexual compatibility	1	2	3	4	5
Harmonious temperament	1	2	3	4	5
Understands you	1	2	3	4	5
Wants what you want	1	2	3	4	5
Shares your passions and worldview	1	2	3	4	5

Kindness	1	2	3	4	5
Charming	1	2	3	4	5
Physically attractive	1	2	3	4	5
Generous	1	2	3	4	5
Easygoing	1	2	3	4	5
Socially polished	1	2	3	4	5
Understands your rhythms	1	2	3	4	5
Sense of humor	1	2	3	4	5

Chapter Two

Celebrity Encounters

Celebrity encounters tend to be among the desirable types of erotic dreams. These are typically fulfillment dreams and fantasies, although they can sometimes yield more than transitory pleasure. The types of fantasies we create and the dream situations that throw us together with celebrity lovers can sometimes provide clues to connections and pleasures that are well within our reach.

Tom Cruise Really Loves Me

Before the breakup of Tom Cruise and Nicole Kidman, one woman had a recurring dream that Tom Cruise would come to her, confess that he was no longer happy with his wife, but in fact could no longer conceal that he had a deep passion for *her*. She would waver awhile because he was married, but would then give in, and they would have a wonderful erotic encounter made all the more glorious because of the revelatory-passion element. Even though she had this dream repeatedly over the course of a year, perhaps once a month, each time was completely new, as if Tom had never showed up before and disclosed his secret passion. This is one of the fairly typical celebrity-encounter dreams; we don't like to be confined by probabilities or realism, we want the goods, the real feelings, and the dream guy all in one swoop.

In the background was the fact that the woman didn't really have a crush on Tom Cruise in waking life; she was sort of neutral about him, depending on the role he played and the film he was in. She was in a relationship that was pretty sound and didn't leave her feeling lonely or unattended. Both of those factors made it a bit less likely that this dream was exclusively her mind's attempt to fulfill a fantasy. Then we considered what made the dream so hot? If it wasn't the guy involved, or just having some great sex, then why was it so memorable, and more important, why was it a recurring theme?

Recurring themes tend to be personal, unique, and meaningful. We all may have a dynamite sex dream once in a while in which we borrow a celebrity for a night, if we're lucky. But when the psyche selects the same person to play that role repeatedly in the same type of pattern, it's more than just random luck or sexy fun.

What made the dreams work for this woman was the surprise factor. That is perhaps also why, although she had many Cruise encounters where he essentially behaved the same way, she was shocked anew each time he professed his feelings for her. Then of course, she would realize she felt the same way, only she'd never consciously thought of it until he told her how he felt. So essentially, these dreams went to a lot of trouble to set the stage for that rush of erotic recognition, in which a previously neutral person is suddenly revealed as *hot* and you then can't get each other's clothes off fast enough. Also the dreams went to a lot of trouble to create a high level of emotional disclosure and preamble. Not only are these erotic dreams, but there is all this explanation about how he doesn't love his wife, he really loves the dreamer, and he can't bear any longer to do without her. Even the dreamer thought this was pretty unnecessary for a good sex dream—why did her mind put all that in there? She described herself as being just as able to do it on the kitchen table in her dreams as the next person; it really wasn't necessary to put in all that undying love stuff to make it okay for her to have an encounter with him. As we explored these facets of the dream, it began to emerge that these dreams were indeed like movies. On one level the obvious story was about unrequited passion breaking through into nice, sweaty sex. On another level, though, we wondered if the dreams were tracing the shape of a question that her psyche was struggling with, and recurring in response to her inner stirrings.

Look at how she eventually paraphrased the dream and stepped back to make generalizations about it. "Tom Cruise is someone I admire most for being an artist who has made a huge success and acquired power in the real world. He comes to me and says he's come to a realization about his partnership, it doesn't satisfy him, and his passion is for me. I then recognize my passion is for him." We then wondered what message, if any, was imbedded in this theme. She was a counselor who longed to use her artistic talent, but who never really created any art because it wasn't commercially viable. Since the erotic pulse of the dreams centered around the explosion of recognition, the "shock of surprise and desire," we wondered if there was some truth about her art and her power that she was largely unaware of in the day-to-day course of things. As we discussed this possibility, she felt we were on to something. She really did hunger most for a way to express her talents and also to have some kind of recognition or validation for creative work. This might help explain why her psyche chose Tom Cruise to star as the surprise lover in the dreams. He wasn't her erotic choice of fantasy lover, he was an exemplar of someone who took his talents as they were and found vehicles for their expression in highly successful ways.

Partially in response to this series of dreams, she began looking into programs and credentials in art-therapy fields, which combine creative work with therapeutic modalities of healing, support, and teaching. Perhaps there will be a way for her to connect artistry with business, expression with service. This type of romantic erotic dream is a good example of the psyche's urging to integrate rather than fragment your gifts and to find a way to share them with others.

Waking Up Too Soon

To the disappointment of many, one typical variety of celebrity-laden erotic dream appears more directed to the promise of a sexual encounter than to the detailed action (one hopes) will follow. In this scenario you're thrown together by circumstance with a favorite celebrity, your eyes lock and you both know you're going to slip away together and consummate the scorching chemistry swirling between you. It's one of those dizzying times when almost anywhere will do, and the world slides away suddenly insignificant as you get lost in sensation. Just as it seems the two of you will surely catch on fire, you simply *wake up*. No no no! You wiggle into your mattress and try to crawl back into sleep, back into the dream, and back into his arms. Usually, though, it's just gone.

Why does this happen? One explanation is the same reason why we sometimes wake up before we hit the ground in a falling dream: We get too excited! When heart rate, respiration, and blood pressure rise, in some cases we essentially wake ourselves up.

Over the years, though, I've begun to believe that at least some of these dreams present exactly as they are supposed to. That is, we aren't awakening prematurely; we are instead mirroring precisely what we are doing with some aspect of waking life. The shape of these dreams is recognition, desire, impulsive acceptance of what you want, and then a shift of consciousness so abrupt it cuts you off completely from the richness of the experience. It may sound abstract, but this is indeed a pattern that manifests to some extent as women approach intense passion, power, or a sense of destiny. It is unclear to what extent this is universal, or what the source of this pattern may be. Yet in talking with women over the years about their passions, dreams, and desires, I've noticed a kind of reflexive recoil that occurs: Often the closer we get to what we want, the more likely we are to do a sudden shift that stops us short of the finish line or "forces" us to abandon our passion when it is finally within reach. The more intense, heartfelt, or central the passion, the more likely we are to experience weird "misfortune" or challenges, either internal or external, that seem to be like a magnetic force trying to push us away from fulfillment.

This certainly does not imply that there's no way around this phenomenon. On the contrary, knowing that there is a certain riptide that may try to pull you away from your goal is often all it takes to break the spell. If you have been having some of these abrupt awakening erotic dreams, consider whether they may, in one sense, be reflecting a kind of snap-back phenomenon in your real life, either around sexuality or in the broader sense around any kind of passion or power.

Stand-in Stars

One of the reasons celebrities crop up in erotic dreams so frequently is that they are identified with particular qualities. Celebrities are like billboards for certain qualities with which they are publicly identified. Perhaps one reason why many stars become stars is that something about them stirs our tendency to project onto them. While many celebrities are just plain gorgeous, some have rather complex qualities that strike a chord with the dreamer. If you're not clear about why a certain celebrity is starring in your erotic dreams, consider what qualities they represent in their broad public personae and what they represent to you.

Think about it this way: Which celebrities, if any, do you feature in your fantasies, while making love, masturbating, or just whiling away your time? Are these the same sex stars that appear in your dreams? Probably not. Here's an example. One woman fantasizes about Russell Crowe. He strikes her as unapologetically masculine, kind of rough, and unpredictable.

The sort of man that can shake you out of your need to enter data into the computer and turn things upside down for a while. He's like a masculine storm front that can make even the most exhausted, neutral professional woman feel very female indeed. Perhaps for these reasons, as well as others, Mr. Crowe appears to be a very popular "borrowed" fantasy figure. This same woman, however, tends to have erotic dreams about Hugh Grant.

This reflects one of the differences between our daytime fantasies and our dreams. Fantasies indulged in during sex or masturbation tend to be high-stimulation, high-arousal selections designed to heighten excitement and bring on orgasm. The stars of our dream encounters are often more complex and may represent qualities in ourselves, or sides of our current partners. For this woman, Hugh Grant represents sensitivity and humor. These are strong qualities she possesses herself, and she feels this series of dreams is not so much about who she would like to take to bed as much as about the quality she wants to have more of in her life.

Identifying Characteristics

Some celebrities stick in our minds because of a role they have recently played or because we just saw them in a film. But more often we have individual labels or qualities we associate with the celebrity. Remember, your dreaming mind is not concerned with courtesy or political or social correctness. Sometimes dreams borrow a celebrity and exaggerate a quality as if to make a point. To make sense of your dreams, sometimes you need to give yourself permission to analyze them without feeling apologetic about the stereotypes or caricatures the dreaming mind has sketched.

One woman found that her celebrity dreams reflected how she was feeling about her own body and her eating habits. She sometimes used food as a way of coping with stress, and would gain weight and then feel uncomfortable and unhealthy. When this pattern occurred she would tend to have sexual dreams about the late John Candy, Drew Carey, or Marlon Brando. These dreams were not unpleasant, but she wondered at first why she kept having sex dreams about men whom she considered to be overweight. Then it dawned on her that, of course, she was "feeling fat" and thrashing around with her tendency to binge as a relief from stress and as a source of reliable pleasure when she was feeling overworked. These erotic partners were evidently a kind of code for how she felt when she neglected to take care of herself.

Once she understood them, the dreams served as a warning signal that brought her up short and helped her to remember to respond to stress with a more varied approach. Interestingly, too, these stars were men she genuinely liked, and she had often wished they might take greater care of their health, because they were such talented and interesting people. In this sense the dreams may have been more than just warning, because they did not present people she found repugnant or disgusting. Instead there was the sense that these are special men, gifted and talented and worthy of good health. The implication is that this woman likes herself and feels worthy as well.

Archetypal Roles

When a celebrity is in a blockbuster movie, or a film that tells
an epic story, for a few years that celebrity apparently is identified in our minds with the role or the characteristics they
had in that film. For example, when *Titanic* was popular, Leo-
nardo DiCaprio was probably the number-one celebrity in
our dreams. This continued for a few years until he was in
enough other films to presumably become less identified with
the character in that film. Obviously *Titanic* was a tragic love
story, and the lead characters were very sympathetic. DiCaprio
was an ordinary fellow, and a bit of an underdog who emerged
as having superior characteristics to the fancier people around
him. The underdog who morphs into a hero halfway through
a story is an archetypal character, and our minds seem to connect this type of character and carry them into our dreams.
For a few years at least, when we dreamed of underdogs with
lots of potential, ordinary people with magical perception, or
the conflict between expectations and adventures, DiCaprio
was the poster boy in our dreams.

A bit more recently Keanu Reeves became a prominent
dream celebrity when he became identified with his role in the
Matrix movies. He crops up in the dreams of women who report they have never given him a thought by day, but who very
much like the movies and found their premise provocative.
When we are struggling to make sense of the cause and effect
in our lives, the extent to which we create our own destiny and
other metaphysical questions, Keanu is the star of our dreams.

Dream Key #2

Decoding Celebrity Encounters

If you have a celebrity encounter in your dreams, and you aren't sure what to make of it, you can begin by looking at what qualities you identify with that celebrity. There are usually at least four steps to this.

1. What is the person famous for? Acting, music, athleticism? Leadership?

2. If you asked ten people on the street, what quality would they associate with this person?

3. What quality do you associate with them?

4. Is there someone in your life, some quality in yourself, or some energy in your life that you would also label the same way?

Let's work this through with a woman who had an erotic dream about Lance Armstrong.

1. He's an athlete.

2. He's identified globally with beating the odds.

3. She thinks of him as determined and able to actualize his vision.

4. Her boyfriend fits this description.

When analyzed, it turned out that this woman was having a dream encounter with the side of her boyfriend that often bothered her most, because it was his obsessive urge to succeed on a large scale that seemed to pull him away from her. The dream was helpful because it showed her that the drive, clarity, and courage in her guy were much of what made her love him. She decided to trust his process and his disposition rather than pout when she felt neglected. She decided that when someone has a vision that is larger than life and the drive to make it happen, you have to give that space.

CHAPTER THREE

Delicious Recognition

Many of us have had the experience of hooking up with someone we've known for a while, but had not thought of in a sexual way until some lightning bolt struck us. The person you knew as Phil the rumpled and lovable neighbor is suddenly transformed into Phil the God of Sex as you look over at his sleeping figure in wonder. Whatever it is that makes us suddenly fall on someone with stunned recognition and appetite, it apparently is very real. Amazed recognition of passion has long been a prominent theme in women's erotic dreams.

In our dreams, the moment of recognition is much more than romantic fantasy. The sense of recognition is so powerful it seems to blend desire with an otherworldly sense of recognition. These dreams are usually encounters; the person may be someone who exists in real life whom you have not considered in an erotic way, or it may be someone fictional (who unfortunately doesn't exist in real life). But in the dream, the moment of recognition is searing in intensity and usually has both erotic and emotional overtones.

He Gets Me

One dream exemplary of this theme was set in an alpine ski resort. The dreamer, an avid skier, paused on the slope and raised her goggles to rub her eyes. A man stopped beside her, raised his goggles, and began to talk to her in a friendly way about the quality of the snow. They didn't get far into their conversation, though, because as they looked into each other's eyes, *it* happened. There was something like an electric potential that arced between them. This wasn't love at first sight, but it was something instantaneous, like running into an old best friend or an old lover and feeling your body quicken with joy even before you actually put a name to the face. She could feel her blood, her bones, and her crotch singly loudly in an instant. With perfect understanding, they put their goggles on and raced to the bottom of the hill, rushing back to her cabin.

With the magic of dream segues, they were quickly naked without having to fumble with zippers and endless layers of clothes. They apparently made love all day, because in the dream it was then dark except for the light made by the fire. As they stared into each other's eyes, she had the feeling that he somehow understood her and knew her in a way that no one ever had before. This, to her, was the ultimate turn-on.

This dream came at a time when the woman was without a love interest, but it helped her to understand more about what she was looking for, and what she needed to hold her interest. She was athletic and robust, enjoying exercise, sex, and living vigorously. Because of her work she had a tendency to connect with men from her professional life, who often did not have any interest in her hobbies or active lifestyle. They found her heartiness intriguing, but she always had to go off and have her adventures on her own. Not only was this lonely, but she also had the underlying feeling that none of her companions really "got" what she was all about. This dream showed her that for her, sex might be better with someone who shared her vitality and love of activities. Like many active people, she couldn't really explain why moving around in space and doing things made her feel more alive, it just did. Instead of sticking with men who share her professional interests, she is now going to look for companionship among people who share her sense that vitality and sexuality are fed by physical activities. This dream, with its dramatic moment of recognition, seemed to highlight that being with someone equally active and vital would be a deliciously compatible arrangement.

The Man Downstairs

One woman who lived in a two-story home had an intriguing dream that there was a phantom fellow from an alternate dimension living in the downstairs section of her house. In the dream he had been living there for some time. Although she seldom glimpsed him, she began to feel his presence more and more. At first this was frightening, but as she was better able to perceive him, she realized that this was someone who had been around *for years* waiting for her to be able to see him. She became aware that this fellow wanted to have sex with her, because somehow whenever he looked at her, she could also feel him touching her, probing her, and fondling her with his mind.

He was sort of attractive in an amorphous way, like looking at a handsome man through a fog. She tried to stay away from him because she was unsure what this whole thing was about. She would withdraw and go upstairs, because somehow the dimension he lived in only overlapped the downstairs portion of the house. As some dreams do, this one seemed to bridge an extended time span, and still within the dream, she couldn't sleep for feverishly thinking about the man downstairs. When she finally gave up and raced downstairs, she found him standing at the foot of the stairs waiting for her. When they came together, it was not only sexy, but otherworldly as well. They floated to the couch and landed gently on it as he touched her reverently but also possessively. She found herself vibrating with a strange excited hum. His hands, mouth, and penis not only *seemed* to be everywhere at once, they *were* everywhere: Evidently he could be in more than one place at the same time in his dimension. Their coming together made the air crackle. In the dream they seemed to go on endlessly, floating from place to place, position to position, as if he had been waiting many lifetimes for her to glimpse him, and now that she had, all the pent-up passion was going to be played out.

Despite the surreal and otherworldly quality of this dream, the dreamer said that when she awoke the next morning, she lay in bed and stared at the ceiling in a daze. She also had the most palpable feeling that she truly could not be sure whether or not it had been a dream. What would she find when she went downstairs? Seemingly, it was a dream, but what a dilly of an erotic-recognition dream.

This erotic hangover is one of the hallmarks of an erotic-recognition theme. On a visceral level you awaken stunned that you've just had the best sex of your life, or been known and explored and shared at a deeper level than ever before. In the first moments of consciousness, the fact that it was in a dream seems less important than the fact that it *happened* and you want to absorb it and savor it. The intensity of these experiences isn't really made less by the realization that it was a dream. Some women tell me they have stumbled through the better part of a day in a sexual hangover, unable to think about much beside their recent experience. Instead of being "unreal," these dreams often seem *more real* than waking reality, although this is incredibly difficult to explain or understand if you haven't had such a dream.

As is often the case, the dream of the man downstairs came at a time when the dreamer was without a partner, and when she was so busy she was not thinking in terms of sex or relationships. On one level we could assume that when we're alone, perhaps sexually hungry, our dreams might rise to the occasion and provide some kind of fun once in a while. This is certainly possible; anyone who has followed a strict diet for a while will notice that they start to dream about delicious food. But identifying the trigger for a dream or the sensation or stimuli that gave rise to it isn't quite the same as interpreting what it contains or implies.

This woman believes that the man downstairs represents a side of her that is more passionate and mysterious than her everyday self. Ultimately the detail and the extraordinary qualities of the dream just do not add up to it being a sexual snack to tide her over until the real thing comes along. She also finds comfort in the fact that in the dream she found love "right under her nose." This dream, like almost all erotic-recognition themes, underscores the intoxicating quality of feeling known, recognized, and touched on some essential level.

The 30/70 Rule

While every dream, and every dreamer, is unique, I work from the presumption of the 30/70 rule. Here is how it works. When evaluating the meaning of a dream for what merit or significance it may have, it seems that 30 percent of what is going on in a dream has to do with your physiology, your environment, or recent stimuli. You may dream about George Clooney because you just saw him in a movie that night. That's the 30 percent. But what you do with George, and what your mind does with the dream, is the other 70 percent. Two people who go to the same movie, who borrow the same movie star, will have two very different dreams. The trigger or stimulus is the same, but the text of the story and the variables involved are purely your own.

Many things contribute to our dreams, including how our bodies feel and what our hormones are up to. For example, are you ovulating or getting your period? You may feel more or less sexy than usual, more attracted to sexual partners or more annoyed with them in different points in your cycle. Did you eat too much or take cold medicine? Heavy physical feelings can contribute to nightmarish twists in dreams, and medications can tinge our dreams with a macabre or feverish quality.

Did you need to use the bathroom and refuse to awaken? Some of our never-getting-to-use-the-toilet dreams arise in the background of a full bladder sending repeated signals your way. If your bedroom was freezing and the covers fell off, you might find your dream suddenly shifts to a campground in Alaska even though you've never been there.

The way your body feels, the immediate environment, and recent stimuli tend to kick in or set your dreams in a certain direction. But that is only about 30 percent of the story. The rest is all you: your feelings, your fantasies and fears, the current chapter you're living in your life, and maybe what you need to make you feel known, appreciated, and loved.

Who Knows Where or When

Déjà vu is a controversial topic and none of us is really sure how it works. It is the sensation that what is happening has already happened once; you have either dreamed the moment you are now living, or you've been through it before somehow. One thing is for sure, many women have found themselves in relationships that didn't exactly add up or pass their criteria, but which they found irresistible because of the powerful sense that they already knew and were connected to the other person.

One woman launched into an important relationship to explore the undeniable recognition she felt with a man she met in a seminar. Although their relationship was not lifelong, it was a positive experience, and it served to deepen her certainty that something about that déjà vu experience was very real. They were thrown together by an exercise that involved one person sitting quietly with their eyes closed while the other person told a story. She sat quietly and listened to the story. When she opened her eyes and looked into his, the room literally tipped for a second, and her visual field seemed to ripple. She knew she had lived that very moment with this man before. She knew his voice, his gaze, his hands, his smell. Like most of us, she had nowhere to take that realization, and it seemed silly to interrupt him to say, "We've done this before!" She didn't say anything, but she did accept his invitation when he eventually asked her out, and they had a marvelous love affair. Years later she continues to fantasize, not about the man as you might expect, but about the moment of recognition that made the room ripple and the floor tilt.

We never know when we're going to have a moment of déjà vu, and we never know how real it is or how much credence to give it. I think, though, that it is an anomalous phenomenon that can serve to remind us of an important principle. The subjective sense of recognition, of knowing someone, or of being known is one of the deepest of our relational experiences; we crave it emotionally, sexually, and spiritually.

Elevator-Phobia Therapy

One woman who had a mild fear of elevators would often dream of riding an elevator and panicking whenever she was in a stressful period of her life. Typically the elevators behaved with psychotic whimsy, traveling too fast up or down or sideways, and failing to respond to her careful floor selections.

One night, however, she had a dream that seemed to combine erotic fantasy with therapy in a way that only Hollywood and our dreams can seem to pull off.

In the dream she got into an elevator with a handsome man who was played by Bruce Willis. (He wasn't a movie star in the dream, he was just a guy on the elevator, but the part was played by Mr. Willis.) She pushed a button, and the elevator started to rise too high. She started to feel a wave of fear, a sense that she might panic or go out of control. She just popped across the elevator and grabbed the man and held on. He seemed unsurprised and stroked her hair. "Nervous?" he asked softly. She nodded. "Well, maybe we can give you something else to think about." He then lifted her chin and smiled at her in a teasing familiar way, as if they had been friends and naughty lovers for years. She recognized him, although she couldn't remember how they knew each other. He kissed her for the longest time, and the vertigo and panic were replaced by a welcoming feeling of lazy heat. Somehow the elevator didn't move, and they took all the time they wanted to have sex against the walls with her legs wrapped around him. She smiled to herself even in the dream, thinking this would make a memory that she could take with her from now on as she rode on elevators.

Prior to the dream, she had seen an old movie in which Bruce Willis had played some kind of psychotherapist treating a group of people who were getting murdered one by one. The subplot of the movie involved his affair with a mysterious young woman and some intriguing sex scenes. The dreamer thought probably Bruce Willis was chosen to play the starring role in her elevator dream because he was now recently associated in her mind with therapy and with sex. This dream did give her something new to think about as she rides elevators, and perhaps the other people wonder why she is smiling.

Dream Key #3

The Gift of Recognition Themes

Though they may appear complex, sometimes dreams come to help us simplify our process. Erotic-recognition dreams are good examples of this simplicity. Here is a list of reasons why we may have these types of dreams. See if any of these points apply to you.

1. You will know what you want and who you want when you see it. You don't have to worry and overanalyze every little nuance of behavior or try to change people who just aren't right for you. Relax and trust your core to resonate with recognition when it's right.

2. You have more facets of strength, talent, courage, and communion than you know. Once in a while you collide with a situation, a person, or a dream that practically screams at you to acknowledge and *recognize* yourself as more. Most people aren't in denial about their problems; they are in denial of their gifts and their *bigness*. It isn't bragging if you just hold more space for yourself and let your life get a little bit bigger.

3. For some, being with someone is not enough. If you are the kind of person who is not easily known, and you're with someone who cannot seem to get what you're all

about, it can be lonely even though you're not alone. One thing that may help is to trade a book with someone you care about. Pick a book that describes your experience or means something to you, and have your partner read it. Let your partner pick a book that means something essential to him, and you read it. If you just wave a book at someone, you'll notice it is still sitting on the coffee table three years later, untouched. But trading a book can work; give it a try.

CHAPTER FOUR

Ideal Situations

While erotic dreams often contain elements of trouble that interfere with pleasure, probably reflecting the actual complexity of women's lives, some of our dreams are sheer delight. Interestingly, these dreams often involve extraordinary situations or settings. The partners or sex stars of these dreams sometimes appear almost secondary to the bliss of being in a setting that ignites feelings or transforms perception.

Sex on the Home Planet

One woman told me that her best erotic dream took place in a setting that was a recurring one in her dreams. From time to time, say once a year, she dreams she is visiting her home planet; that, although she is human, she is actually from another place. In these dreams she magically returns to her true home, a beautifully lit, softly spacious planet with two moons. This planet is all silver and gentle light, and there is a home on the beach that has open walls because the temperature is so forgiving. In these dreams she stays at this home for a rest, saturating herself with the feeling of spaciousness, bathing her senses in the gentle temperature, soft winds, and silvery light.

In one of these dreams there was a man in the house, and while she was there they had sex; which was, and was not, like earthly sex. Somehow there was not the separation of roles, or the sensation of the difference between male and female that we take for granted on Earth. Instead, they were more similar than dissimilar, and when they caressed each other, light wafted out from their bodies, shimmering where their skin touched. Every contact by finger or lips was in itself intercourse. The exchange of essence and charge between them was ongoing, rather than occurring at a point of climax. At one point she looked up and saw there was a matrix of light above them, lifting and intertwining like smoke from a fire, but luminous and dancing like the Northern Lights. As they merged, the atmosphere around them was enhanced and enriched as if the molecules of the air became compatible with each other. Sex was not merely a pleasure; it was a making-better of the surroundings as well. As you can imagine, these home-planet dreams are incredibly restoring to this dreamer, and the elements involved in her idyllic love scene do suggest qualities that honor the ordinary life as well.

I love the idea of having a "home planet," a place that is your natural habitat, which nourishes and supports you, and frees you from tension and the pervasive amnesia of daily life, the amnesia that makes you forget you are sensual, forget you are spiritual, forget your flashes of brilliance. Think about this for a moment: What would your home planet be like? The pace, the colors, the climate, all can tell you something about what you would find nourishing in your current environment.

This dreamer is an unusual person, and as such, possibly often feels like a fish out of water. Her sensual dream suggests that for her, sex represents an opportunity for almost spiritual communion. The dream also hints that she may consider her actions to have rippling effects impacting elements that most of us would consider entirely separate from her. Yet this is not a planet with a lot of bells and whistles, is it? This is a place of serene temperate breezes and houses without walls. It is open, safe, and magically transformative.

It is worth remembering that whatever heaven we may dream is also somehow within us. The essence is available as a set of feelings and experiences. Space, privacy, room to be herself, and awareness of mystical or metaphysical nuances appear to be part of this dreamer's ideal setting. Any situation or partner with room for these qualities will likely lift her up and help re-create the feelings of paradise.

The Flamenco-Tango

Dancing is a frequent image in dreams dealing with sexuality. In some of these dreams, no overt sex occurs, but then, it almost does not need to.

A woman who was in the process of falling in love had a dream that she was a flamenco dancer, performing an exciting and fiery dance amidst a group of people. Although she had short dark hair in waking life, in the dream, her hair cascaded down her back and flew out as she spun around. Her gown was red, full-skirted, and slit so that her legs were unrestrained. A man from the crowd joined her in the dance, and the music shifted to a tango. She wrapped one leg around his back, and they rippled as if their bodies were a single form. People in the crowd were stomping their feet or clapping to the beat as the woman and her partner moved sensuously around with abandon. They moved so well their eyes were closed some of the time, the music running up their spines and causing them to dip and bend. Always their torsos were pasted together, their movements a single expression. As the dream ended she had wrapped her legs around his back and was hanging over backward, her hair brushing the floor as he moved in a smooth circle.

It is not unusual for women who do not dance in waking life to be incredible dancers in their dreams. It is also fairly typical when having a dream about freedom and sensuality to have long wild hair that blows in the wind like a horse's mane. This dream appears to be a celebration dance expressing the chord of passion struck in her new relationship. The woman feels exotic, reckless, capable, and well matched. In this dream, as in other idyllic settings, the lovers are supported, accepted, and applauded by their environment. This dream is warm and earthy, and pulsates with undiluted feelings. Yet part of what may make this possible is the setting. This dance does not occur in a vacuum. It is part of a gathering, performed to perfectly sensual music in a gown that does not confine the dreamer. There is a sense of freedom supported by an environment that celebrates expression. Certainly there is also implied trust in the partner, since she winds around him like a snake and hangs upside down with complete freedom. She can assume any position, make any move, and disregard gravity.

Ideal settings make possible the suspension of normal concerns and barriers to feeling. There is a perfect flavor of wildness here, but it is wildness in the background of acceptance and trust.

The Hometown Tryst

In the Pacific Northwest, where I live, many people have moved to Portland or Seattle from surrounding rural areas. Our memories of early life involve landscapes that are rural and simple; our relationships to those memories seem to evolve over time. Having escaped the early mud on my shoes to live in the city, I now hunger to return to a home in the woods. It seems that whether literal or symbolic, the "return" to home, and to acceptance of the past, is part of life's journey.

Some dreams combine the theme of going home with surprising eroticism; we return to find the thing we left in search of long before.

One woman dreamed that she was visiting her hometown for a kind of festival, like a rodeo or a country fair. As she walked behind the bleachers, she encountered a young man who remembered her from their childhood. She did not remember him, or only vaguely. But they leaned against the stands and talked for quite a while as twilight closed in. Voices died down, and they were more and more alone. They embraced, and he kissed her with a thoroughness that surprised and excited her. She had forgotten that a kiss could rock you back like that. They were between a wooden fence and the back of the bleachers, and they shifted slightly so that her back was to the fence. She leaned back against it, and they had sex standing up. Her mind flickered to wonder if anyone would happen by, but no one did, and soon she was not thinking at all.

This setting is very simple, as is the action of this dream. A woman visiting home has a surprisingly nice, almost adolescent tryst against a fence at a country fair. Youngsters who grow up in small towns tend to find modest corners behind buildings or beneath bleachers to steal away and explore each other. Interestingly, this dream seems to find that early hideaway still very sexy. She is surprised that a simple kiss can be so "thorough" and rock her back. This hints that perhaps part of her is realizing that variety and complexity are not necessary to her own sensual nature. The visceral connection she makes with this childhood acquaintance suggests that she may discover that what she wants is simpler than she realized. In a mythic psychological sense, when we turn back toward what we discarded earlier in life, and pick it up and see it as valuable, it is then that we really begin to be more free and to get more traction with fulfilling our dreams. Whether this dream is truly about her sex life, or more globally about her plans for the future, a dream of "the return" is almost always a marker of maturity and clarity.

As a sexual setting, this country fair is modest and simple, but again, it is safe and supportive. If someone happened by while they were banging against the fence, that person would probably just chuckle and wander off. The dream seems to hint that gut-level connection is more sensual than sophisticated banter, that twilight behind the bleachers in your hometown may be transporting, and surprisingly satisfying.

In the Meadow

A favorite dream one woman shared with me was of her erotic encounter with a freckled man. Although in waking life she is a brunette, in her dream, she had long red hair worn loosely, and her skin was covered with freckles.

The dream took place outdoors, in a meadow near a small pond. A redheaded man approached her and took her hand. They ran to a nearby tree, where he had spread a blanket on the ground. There, they laughingly took their clothes off and made love, finding delight in their mutual freckles and pale skin. It was as if they shared a secret the rest of the world would not understand, and they found this funny and delightful. Their bodies fit together perfectly, and their laughter turned to gasps of passion. At some point after they finished making love, the dreamer thought to herself: *How could I ever have thought my freckles were ugly?*

She awoke the next morning with a sense of well being and relaxation and wondered about the dream. Clearly it was a fun and lighthearted sex dream, and she awoke with a smile on her face. But what about those freckles and the outdoor setting? When our dreams take departures from our waking lives and give us pleasure in doing so, the implication is that some quality in the dream might also please us in our regular lives.

Neither she nor her real-life partner look anything like those two, and they don't make love outside. They are admitted perfectionists. As we explored the dream, it became apparent that one of the most important qualities of the dream was the red-haired, freckled quality of the two lovers. The dreamer said she tended to groom herself often, scrutinizing her appearance for any "flaws." While Hollywood and advertisers seem to encourage us to strive for an airbrushed appearance, this can be a somewhat numbing practice over time. While we may want to be attractive in service of love and sex, paradoxically the reflex of separating the self into acceptable and unacceptable parts is deadening. Sometimes the threads of this practice weave into a fabric of compulsiveness rather than aliveness.

The randy freckled couple seemed to revel in their spots and to find a blanket under a tree, the perfect place to enjoy each other. In the dream the freckles were not flaws, they were punctuation marks of individuality which she and her fictional lover had in common. Also, and perhaps most important, her dream had concluded with a clear thought: How could she have thought her freckles were ugly? When a dream contains a clear quotation, it may be revelatory. For her, the question roughly translated to: "Why do I think the things that make me individual are flaws to be concealed?"

This question, posed after a fulfilling session of lovemaking with a partner who was also covered with freckles, gave her an important idea. The pursuit of perfection, in appearance, grooming, possessions, and lifestyle, can backfire on us by making our spotty, spicy qualities seem unfit for consumption. What if she and her partner spent less time avoiding flaws and more time comparing freckles? She felt that one of the qualities missing in her life was the freedom and secret joy she had felt as the wild redhead in the dream. It would never have occurred to her redheaded alter ego to worry about flaws or the fact that her hair was hopelessly tangled, first by wind and later by passion.

The perfect setting here is made possible by acceptance of

uniqueness, and by finding joy in sharing that uniqueness. Perhaps this simple blanket in a meadow hints that the dreamer will find bliss, not in constructed perfection, but in the recognition of a different kind of perfection that already exists in her and around her.

Dream Key #4
Cultivating Ideal Settings

The qualities that make our ideal erotic settings perfect can often teach us something about what nourishes us, both sexually and in a more general sense as well. Did you find as you read these women's dreams that you could enter one of these dreams and almost drink up the space, the music, or the warmth of that setting? Were you reminded of a dream of your own, or a favorite sensual scene from a movie unforgettable to you, because it was so sensual you practically melted into your seat? If you recall a dream or a scene that was ideal to you, make some notes in your journal about what was most delicious to you.

Setting
People and environment
Your qualities (hair, clothes, other)
The partner's qualities

Most of us think we already know what is attractive to us, what is fun and appealing. Yet dreams often point out things we not only don't think about, but would *never* imagine, such as the perfectionist who came to wonder whether embracing "flaws" might be sexier than constantly tweezing her life away. We also fail to register qualities in the environment that are sexy and liberating to us. Below are some attributes for you to consider in terms of how they make you feel. Consider those that resonate for you and make a mental list of what pleases you so that you can re-create them when possible, in your intimate life, and also when you need to restore your energy.

Solitude
Select people around or nearby
Familiar setting
Exotic setting
Earthy and visceral ambience
Rarefied, mystical, or metaphysical setting
Removed from daily routine
Planned and known time schedule
Unplanned, swept away
Slow, unhurried connection
Sudden impulsive passion
Soft light, hazy edges
Nighttime
Twilight
Broad daylight
Sense of open space
Sense of privacy, shelter
Outdoors
Indoors
Complexity
Simplicity

Now write down the qualities that you choose in a single line so that you can see them together and begin to get a picture of your ideal erotic environment. If there are some qualities that were not listed above, that you now realize, be sure to include them. The next time you are going to be intimate, or masturbate or restore your energy, try to put some of these qualities in place to the extent that it is possible.

PART TWO

Sorting Dreams

CHAPTER FIVE

The Old Flame

One of the questions I'm asked most frequently is why we continue to dream of people we have not seen in years. Are these dreams revealing that you still carry a torch for your high-school sweetheart, or that you have unresolved issues with your ex?

For whatever reason, most old-flame dreams tend to be about relationships and sexuality, rather than about the person who stars in them. You will always have a tendency to have dreams about the first person you had sex with, the first person you loved deeply, as well as your most recent relationship. In our dreams people from our sexual history tend to be like commemorative stamps that represent certain types of relationships. Sometimes the greatest lovers turn out to be lousy partners, and after the inevitable sad ending to the relationship, that person gets indoctrinated into the "heartache hall of fame" in your history.

Sex with the Dirty Dog

One woman had a wild and short-lived relationship with a fellow who turned out to be a bit of a bad apple. She survived the fling, but was kind of stung by how nasty things turned out toward the end. However, during their time together, they did have great sex and chemistry that seemed to always be sparking. She came to think of and refer to this fellow as "the dirty dog." It took her awhile to get past the bad taste of this encounter, but eventually she was ready to get close to someone again. However, as she geared up to have a new relationship, she started to have sexual dreams about the relationship she regretted. Why was this happening? She certainly wanted no part of that fellow, nor of anyone like him, sparks or no sparks.

The dreams were not so much about the *person* in her past, as they were about the confusing mix of sex and affection, and risk and benefits of intimacy. Some of our sexual dreams are attempts to make sense of the landscape of relationships, desires, and fears. When hurt feelings get mixed up with intimacy, sex, and desire, there is a sort of post-traumatic stress that kicks up as we approach the territory of love and sex again. It's important to pay attention to the dreams you have as you begin a new relationship or become sexually active again after a respite.

This woman decided that her "dirty dog" dreams were her mind's way of showing her the scars on her heart. In a sense the dreams were simply saying: proceed with caution and stay awake this time. To her this meant two things: staying alert for signs of incongruity in her partner, and staying alert for signs of extravagant compromise in herself. Thus armed, she embarked on a lovely relationship that has so far brought her only happiness and affection.

When we dream of people from the past who wounded us or who contributed to confusion about the results of passion, it may be the psyche's way of helping us remember to take precautions with our lives and with our hearts. But other memories are far sweeter and less contaminated with mixed results.

Touchstones of Passion

Some people from the past are like emblems of passion and discovery. When these characters frequent your dreams their presence may be a signal that in some way you are moving toward passion or connection in a new way.

One woman had an employer who was never a lover in real life, but there was a recognition between them, an understanding. He was the first person who encouraged her talents and her quick mind, and the fact that there was a pull of attraction between them made the connection more profound. Long after she moved on to other jobs and other bosses, she often had erotic dreams of this man, in which he encouraged her spirit while he delighted in her body. For her he combines physical attraction with psychic recognition; for whatever reason, they *saw* each other and celebrated each other's abilities even though they did not have a physical relationship. In her dreams they are always in bed, and there is no plot involved except that they are finally getting to enjoy each other thoroughly. He is as he always was, encouraging her, knowing her, and brushing away her self-doubts. At the same time he functions as a sexual ideal, he also seems to carry the energy of the psychic *encourager*. I believe that just as we all have "inner critics" whose voices contaminate our processes, we also have internal encouragement that can bolster courage or remind us of our purpose.

Interestingly, she usually has these dreams when she is at low points in life or has encountered some kind of roadblock. These dreams serve not only to leave her glowing from a delicious encounter, they also give her a much-needed increase in confidence.

These types of dreams are more than just compensatory: They can be like infusions of positive energy that can carry us forward. They are more than just fun for the night to break up a dry spell; they are emotional, sexual, and psychological fuel that can be highly restorative and lasting.

When we are under stress, we tend to lose track of ourselves and become fragmented. Have you ever gotten together with old friends and found yourself laughing and carrying on, and then left thinking, "Why don't I goof around like that anymore, When did I get so serious?" For myriad reasons, life tends to scatter our powers and fragment our dispositions. Dreams tend to help us put ourselves back together by integrating our facets and helping us feel whole again. I believe that erotic dreams of encounters with encouraging people are the psyche's way of regrouping our forces and renewing our misplaced enthusiasm.

Marking an Era

Just as some people become identified with qualities such as intense sex, emotional betrayal, or encouragement, other people from our past become markers for a particular time in our lives. The high-school sweetheart not only represents a relationship, he also represents that entire chapter in your life: the person you were and the patterns of interaction you had at that time.

One woman often dreams of a short disastrous marriage she had early in life. She was so young and eager to please that she went along with all sorts of poor decisions and grand schemes. Many years later, when she is being passive or too reticent, she will dream that she is again in that marriage. For her, this has nothing to do with the man himself; she has lost touch with him and seldom gives him a thought. But when she is *being the person she was during that chapter of her life* she will again dream of being with that man. These dreams have proven so reliable as markers of this pattern for her that she will immediately sit down and consider where she needs to be more assertive, realistic, or purposeful in her current circumstances.

Dreams about people we have not seen in years or decades seldom have much to do with the character in the dream. Often these dreams are emblematic of patterns in present circumstances that were pronounced during an earlier chapter in our lives.

Recommendations for Current Connections

Even when we dream of the past, we do so in service of the present and future. There is something to learn, to be nourished by, or warned of in our dreams. With the exception of very singular post-traumatic nightmares, our looks into the past are ultimately attempts to help our current lives flourish. This is never more true than when we dream about sex and love.

Conception

A women told me that she believes she knew the night she was conceiving her son, because not only was it a night of perfect passion between her and her husband, but she also felt a kind of rushing of energy, as if she had opened to some cosmic wind and it had entered her. Though her description sounds remarkable, she proved to be correct and has never forgotten the experience. Shortly after her son was born, she and her husband divorced. She said that they had a good physical relationship, and a kind of intangible bond that she could not resist, but that ultimately their relationship did not work, like a table that only has three legs and is never balanced. She wonders now if perhaps they were together at that time so that her son could be born. In any event, she cannot regret that relationship and does not spend much time looking back on it.

At various junctures in her life, she has dreamed of that night, and of some magical wind blowing through her and into her to lodge inside and mysteriously grow. In these dreams she feels the sense of sexual joy, and even more keenly at times, the sense of promise, richness, and contentment. Although she has never had another child, she does have many "creations," in a sense, because she is an artist. She says that when she is stuck on something, one of her erotic-conception dreams will sometimes help her let go and surrender to the process. For her they are a lovely reminder of the way life comes to us, moves through us, and then expresses itself. When she is most content with her work, she feels like a birthing is occurring. When she loses her way and thinks it is about her reputation, her track record, or the opinions of critics, it becomes mechanical and less meaningful.

Prescription Kisses

One woman who worried that her current relationship was getting stale dreamed of visiting a sex therapist with her old boyfriend. In the dream this therapist was pretty progressive (or weird) and insisted that she and her boyfriend have sex on the couch while he watched their technique. Self-conscious and not very into it, they managed to have sex while the therapist occasionally called out encouragement and direction. He had them try a few different positions, which were gymnastically challenging but not very erotic. Finally the session was over, and they felt closer just for having gone through the strange little adventure together. They held hands and sat together on the couch while the therapist made some notes. Finally he tore off a prescription pad and handed it to them. The prescription read: *Spend more time kissing*.

As we discussed the dream, the woman said that she felt

she and her partner might benefit more from situations and gestures of closeness than from trying so hard to turn each other on. The old relationship had run aground, she said, because she and her partner had taken to sniping at each other and had really been too young to ride out the rough patch. In the language of dreams, kissing represents approval and recognition, so the dream therapist had a pretty good suggestion. In a way the dream said: worry less about performance and focus on appreciating and recognizing each other. The dreamer said she was approaching the same junction in the relationship road with this current partner that she had hit with the old flame when things had begun to unravel. So this dream visit to the sex therapist was perhaps her mind's way of getting her attention and giving a very loving prescription to nurture this partnership along.

Exaggerating to Make a Point

When we get frustrated, lonely, or disappointed, it's easy to get on a roll with our troubles and to feel everything has just gone bad. One way to know you're off balance is to notice how dramatically you describe your problems. Do you remember when your kid sister wouldn't leave the house because she had a pimple? Dreams often make fun of our troubles by reflecting our exaggerations.

A friend and I were recently discussing the mixed bag of becoming middle-aged. We poked fun at our foibles and shook our heads over our vanishing vanities. After the conversation, though, she had a dream that told her to wake up and dust herself off.

In the dream she was visiting a town where an old lover still lives. When they saw each other again, the spark was still there, so they were going to have a night together for old time's sake. As they started making out, one of her knees began clicking. Soon his back went out, and they moved guardedly to the bedroom, but then her hip started aching. One thing after another went wrong as their signs of aging made the ensuing encounter less spontaneous and more awkward. Finally the man pulled back and stated the obvious: "We might as well give up on this; we're way too old to have sex again anyway." This was an exaggeration that made her realize she had been taking this attitude herself. Dreams can make our distortions visible by exaggerating and highlighting them. Like a psychic biofeedback mechanism, our dreams can sometimes help us move in the direction of more choices and greater awareness.

Dream Key #5

Understanding What Old Flames Represent

Here is a list of the things an old flame may represent in your dream:

1. The result of the relationship.

2. The chapter of your life at that time.

3. The patterns and behaviors you engaged in at that time.

4. A kind of decision or emphasis.

5. A quality or trait in a current partner.

Some dreams of old flames tend to show us how something from the past is present in our lives again in a new form, whether this is a warning or a signal of hope is an individual matter. Other dreams of old loves offer us reminders of powers and potentials we have lost in the shuffle. It is important not only to identify what the old flame may represent to you, but also what meaning or gift the dream may have for your present circumstances and for your plans for the future. As in the kissing prescription, do you need to acknowledge and validate your partner more? Or are you getting connected with your inner encourager when you need it most? For some, erotic flashbacks have less to do with actual relationships and more to do with passionate expression, which can be just as sacred in its own way.

CHAPTER SIX

Multiple Partners

For those of use who usually sleep with one person at a time, multiple-partner dreams can be intriguing. One woman I know used to have these dreams not infrequently, and she would bring them apologetically to dream-discussion group, passing out written copies to everyone with apologetic murmurs, such as "I hope this doesn't shock you." On the contrary, a hush would fall over the group as we put down our tea and cookies and whipped out our pens to take notes.

All Among Friends

One woman had an intriguing dream that she was apparently having a three-way arrangement with a woman friend from work and her boyfriend. In the dream she "woke up" to find her girlfriend sitting beside her and rubbing her tummy as if she was a child. This was relaxing and so nice of her. Then the friend slid her hand down her tummy and between her legs and began probing and stroking her. This, too, was *very* relaxing. She didn't really think about it, she just angled her legs open to be helpful. But then her leg banged into her boyfriend, who was evidently in bed with her, too. Her eyes popped open, and he mumbled something as he turned toward her. But he didn't say or do anything much, except to make an *mmm* sound, and to wrap himself around her leg. She could feel his erection pressing into her thigh.

This woman didn't get very far into the action zone, but she was surprised at how *cozy* the dream was. After a moment of concern that her boyfriend might take a dim view of things, she drifted off into a haze of sexy cuddling. She worked in a stressful industry that typically had a lot of ups and downs. Having an ally at work in the form of her friend had made her feel much more confident, and they had a lot of fun together. Her boyfriend was similarly low-key, funny, and warm. For the first time in years she felt supported rather than embattled by her life. The dream hints that everything in her life fits together well; the people who love her are wrapped around her like a blanket.

How Long Has He Been Here?

A recently divorced woman had planned to take her time getting back into the dating scene, but as is often the case, she met someone right away and they quickly moved into Full Blown Romance. It was so good to be on the nice side of love for a change rather than being sad all the time.

One night she dreamed that she was in bed with her new fellow. In the dream she had somehow forgotten the fact that one of her old boyfriends from years ago had been renting a room in her house and had also been sleeping with her. Now he was, for some reason, in bed with both of them, just casually pulling her back into him and fumbling to find the edge of her nightgown and lift it up. Actually, it felt pretty nice, but she looked over at her new guy with horror. How had she forgotten to mention her little arrangement? He sat up in bed, and rubbed his eyes, just as the old friend managed to push his erection inside her. She gasped. "Hey, how long has he been here?" her current boyfriend asked, as if suddenly suspicious about the situation.

She woke up wishing that she could finish this dream, have her new fellow go back to sleep so she could enjoy dream sex with a friend she hadn't seen since long before she was married. Why was she dreaming of that man now, and why was he in bed with her and her new companion?

He was a man who had made her feel free and easy sexually, who warmed her all the time. He was also someone from a time in her life when she had been more sexually active and sure of herself. Her new instant romance was throwing her into a different gear, and though it was great, it was an adjustment. Memories of her times with that man made her smile and think of herself as more of a sexual being. This new chapter in her life was reminding her, "pulling her back" into a sexy feeling and sense of herself. Her dream reminded her that she still *is* that person, and getting reacquainted with her is going to be a lot of fun.

All My Exes in One Bed

Years ago dream researcher Gayle Delaney coined the term "casting-call dreams." This is a not-uncommon multiple-partner dream in which most or all of your former lovers show up in one place. Both men and women have this dream, and it can be a tad unsettling.

A contentedly married woman dreamed that she and her husband had a king-size bed in which they slept with all her ex-lovers at the same time. She mostly just had sex with her husband, although the "boys" often whined like children, and said things like "come *on*," hinting that common courtesy required her to share her favors more uniformly. She was pretty prim about this, though, mostly for the benefit of her husband. Sometimes when she slept, she thought she felt exploring fingers, and hopeful erections, but she chose to ignore them.

This is a pretty typical casting-call dream. Although there is room for a lot of action, the orgies one might find interesting seldom occur. The striking quality of the dream is its presentation. Typically the characters in the dream think nothing of the arrangement, or the coincidence that brought them together. I believe casting-call dreams perform a kind of sexual-emotional synthesis for us by throwing all our experiences into one pot and cooking them. Despite our preoccupation with daily events and our relative certainty that we are fine as we are, the dreaming mind is relentless in scanning our happiness. Our dreams distill the sum of our love lives into some kind of truth at regular intervals in our lives, and this process requires periodic reevaluation and resorting.

The Bookends

Sometimes it's not completely clear where one relationship ends and another begins. Most of us try to keep this straight and to play well with others, but occasionally things do get untidy. One woman was "finishing" with one lover and "beginning" with another when she had a dream that let her know this situation was causing more stress than it was worth.

In the dream she was lying on a bed or couch with her old lover, and together they were reading from the diary of her new lover. She lay back in his arms and they took turns reading aloud. They found this fellow was writing a great deal about her, and in the most glowing terms imaginable. She was like a saint, an angel, warm, beautiful, and full of integrity. She twisted around and told her old lover she didn't want to read any more. It didn't seem right at all. Sleeping with him was one thing, but reading his diary seemed like a terrible betrayal, especially since he obviously thought so highly of her.

It was at that moment that she realized she had fallen in love with the new fellow in truth. As she thought that, he appeared at the foot of the bed, and she slid over to him and embraced him.

If she had been slowly transitioning in her choices, this dream helped to clarify where her feelings lay, at the same time it created a ripple of guilt in her. She had been casually sophisticated in waking life, but the dream had caused her to sit up from her old lover's arms and think, "This isn't right, I don't want to do this." Dreams sometimes help us clarify what we feel, recognize what is important, and choose what is right for us.

Married to Four Brothers

One woman dreamed that she was back in the pioneer days and had married four brothers who lived out West. They all shared her amicably enough, and she found their differences and similarities enjoyable. They lived together in a cabin and worked cooperatively together. She slipped quietly from one man to another at night, and no one seemed to think anything of it. The only rule was not to make too much noise. They were big, strong, masculine fellows, a little rough but not unkind. She liked to sleep with two men in one night, and so she had them on something of a schedule. No one in the settlement seemed to think it was odd, either, and their life together went very smoothly.

This woman was happily involved with someone and her life was moving along smoothly. Having a sexy dream is usually welcome fun, but it seemed odd to have four brother-husbands like that. This dream, though, is about more than fun, or a fictional setting that makes multiple partners acceptable. The woman has a lot of power in this dream, and everything in her life is balanced, natural, relaxed, and humming along. She lives in a "settlement," and everyone shares. It is essentially a dream about contentment and connecting with power in many ways on many levels. She has all these "mates" who are also brothers (images of benign power). She is connected with her inner resources and has easy connection with the people around her. This is a good time in her life.

Sometimes sex in dreams symbolizes connecting with powers and passions you have inside in a very healthy way. It's like having good circulation in your spirit and mind. Being able to reach in and grab your courage, confidence, or imagination when you need it. This sounds a bit like New Age applesauce, but it really isn't; dreams often illustrate how and whether we are accessing our resources effectively. Sometimes they simply remind us of the facets and strengths we may have forgotten we have.

Dream Key #6

Triggers of Multiple-Partner Dreams

1. **Sorting through past partnerships.** Even if you're not in a relationship or are in a settled one, you will periodically go through a period of summarizing what you've learned about love and intimacy. You may also read books or see movies with more sexual themes right now, and take a greater interest in conversations about relationships. This preoccupation won't last forever, and you don't need to feel burdened to come up with any sort of ultimate answer or new policy. Just observe this, register what strikes you, and go with it.

2. **Making current relationship transitions.** If you're in the process of leaving or joining someone, all the old files are going to spontaneously open up in your memory and flow through your dreams like a river. You aren't going crazy, you aren't hung up on the past. Your mind is reflecting and helping you get across the transition safely. Pay attention to intuitive flags in your dreams.

3. **Getting reconnected with your sexual circuitry.** Multiple-partner scenes are kind of liberating, even though

ironically they don't seem to have much detailed sexual action. Just knowing there's a mixed-up arrangement seems to make most women wake up feeling a little wilder. This may be the perfect time for you to remember yourself and think of yourself as sexy.

4. **Connecting with intrapsychic resources.** Some multiple-partner dreams are about the multitude of strengths you have. If you suspect this might be the case, make a point to take up challenges with confidence, and to reach for something you've been wanting.

CHAPTER SEVEN

Sex in Public

If you think of the perfect sexual moment in your past, did it take place in the middle of a school auditorium, up on a stage, or during a board meeting? Just as women dream of danger that is not truly hazardous, we also tend to dream of public encounters that are not embarrassing, just fun.

Although women tend to have more dreams set indoors, we have a great number of *erotic* dreams that take place outside or in public areas. It's as if the proximity of other people adds to the sensation of impulsiveness, that I-just-couldn't-help-it feeling. Also, there is an elusive mythology to sex; we have a sneaking suspicion that there are two types of people, those who are "always doing it," and those who aren't. Pretty much everyone wants to be in the first camp, although the reality seems to be that there are seasons and passages in our lives when we are more sexually active and preoccupied than at other times. We are tolerant of other rhythms in our lives, such as periods when we zero in on creating a family, making money, traveling, education, or being of service. But for some reason

we see our sexual lives as either on or off, without much lee-
way. If you're not someone who is *always* doing it, that means
you've turned into one of those people who *never* does it.
Yikes!

Public-sex dreams are not only fun, they also remind us
that our sexual selves are alive and well, still getting into mis-
chief in surprising ways. Sometimes we just do wild things:
get up on stage with the rock star and *do it* in front of the audience, or pick a public spot for a tryst and then feign shock
when people stumble upon you.

Public-Sex Fantasies

One of the most popular types of fantasies for many involves
some type of public exhibition. Many women fantasize about
being onstage while having sex, or being in an auditorium full
of people. A contemporary version of this fantasy deals with
being the star of an Internet porn site, where you have sex
with a partner and it's carried around the world instantly, presumably to people who watch your every move eagerly. As you
lift up your hips, people around the world groan and reach between their legs. This fantasy involves power, proof of desirability, naughtiness, and of course marks you indisputably as
one of the doing-it, rather than the not-doing-it folks. It's almost as if you have sex once, but it's multiplied by the number
of people who watch and presumably get turned on by you.
This fantasy also offers dual excitement, because the stage set
of the porn site is an encapsulated erotic setting: detached
from normal life and where sex is expected, while the camera
and the Internet provide the exposure and the public proof of

wildness. It is no wonder this is an intriguing variation of the public exposure fantasy.

In our dreams the fantasy also tends to include encapsulation and exposure in a neat way.

The Boondoggle

One woman who often traveled for her job dreamed of having a fling with an attractive coworker. In the dream she and a number of colleagues were off at a resort-type place for a series of meetings and training sessions. The resort had a workout and recreation area adjacent to the pool. She was walking on a treadmill in an appealing outfit when the dishy coworker came in and joined her. He was lifting weights and wearing one of those back-support belts that make people look like Viking warriors. He walked over to her, she stepped off the treadmill, and they grabbed each other. He moved her to a table and she laid back on it, as through dream magic she became naked. They began having sex, with him standing next to the table, as if demonstrating the effectiveness of excellent lumbar support on performance. In the mix at some point they became aware of the glass walls and sliding doors out to the pool area, where numerous people were of course watching the action. Instead of making this a moment to run for cover, the presence of the onlookers intensified the excitement.

This dream combines a number of fantasy elements, including enclosure/exposure. The action begins with privacy; they are the only two people in the gym. Finally they are alone and can steal a few minutes to have at each other. Then of course, they are not alone, but are on display to all their friends. The action is very much in the exhibition mode; she is on a raised table like someone who might be demonstrating a skill at a training seminar. A number of exhibition dreams place the sexual action on a lifted background, a stage, table, or platform of some kind.

This woman derived great satisfaction from her work and enjoyed traveling and being in with the movers and shakers in her department. She also had a sexual crush on the star of this dream, who was married and not a likely candidate for any real-life liaisons. But the dream wrapped up the infusion of personal satisfaction she actually got from work with a fantasy of the fellow who always exuded a frisson of heat as she passed him in the hall.

Far from being embarrassed when the audience is spotted, this dreamer is turned on and driven to continue. While most exhibition dreams involve public display, many of them seem to include the device of the exposure being "accidental" or un-avoidable. Once the lovers become aware they have an audi-ence, they are too involved to care, and often feel a rush of intensified pleasure.

Gourmet Sex

There is a popular television gourmet chef who is funny, charming, and sensual on his show. Sometimes it's difficult to know if the fascination comes from all the ingredients he just threw into the batter, or whether it's *him* we want. The audi-ence frequently moans in an almost sexual way when he adds more spice, cream, or chocolate to the dish.

One woman, who is also something of a gourmet, had an exhibition dream about this TV chef. In the dream, she was visiting him on the set of his show, and they were doing a run-through of some recipe that she had designed and was sharing with him. At one point, as they were discussing "kicking up" the intensity of the recipe, they began kissing and caressing each other. Ingredients notwithstanding, they cleared some counter space, and soon she was up on the counter learning that indeed neither of them had any fear of intensity. She looked up and saw the assorted cameras in the ceiling and corners of the set. She also saw that the cameras were *on*, the little red lights were all lit. As they continued having sex, she also could see herself on television sets everywhere, somehow transmitting their little episode around the world. She did not miss a beat; in fact, the cameras being on seemed to intensify the situation.

This is not only a dream of sexual exhibition, but it's also a dream about connecting with someone who has gained notoriety for a talent the dreamer herself shares. When this occurs, the dreaming mind seems to be doing multiple tasks. It is providing fun and adventure, fulfilling a fantasy. It is also drawing a parallel between the dreamer and the person upon whom she projects her own potentials for external recognition. She knows and loves food, intensity, sensuality, people, and publicity. This does not mean she necessarily should have a cooking show, or be on television, but there is a hint here that what she loves about this TV chef is really already alive and well in her. We are intoxicated with proximity to celebrities in dreams, not only for the obvious thrill involved, but also because symbolically this represents how close we are, and how satisfied we are, when we get in touch with our own unique gifts and abilities.

Most women spend their lives swimming against the current to try to find time to "indulge" their interests or talents. We don't necessarily receive much encouragement for our preoccupations, but instead feel pressures that seem to constantly try to pull us away from our passions. When we connect in dreams with someone who not only gets to express their passions, but also is applauded for them, it is one of the sexiest games in town. I would argue that we are not simply having a wish-fulfillment fantasy about the celebrity in these cases, we are being reminded by the psyche where our "juice" in life lies, and that by moving toward our enthusiasms we may also revitalize all corners of our lives.

Sometimes our dreams seem to be triggered by incidents that get us thinking about sex, or wondering what it would be like to be someone else.

Jacuzzi Froth

One woman who belonged to a health club was there late one night and saw her exercise instructor in the hot tub with one of the male members. It was apparent to everyone in the club that the two were very friendly, but she was a little surprised to note that as they soaked in the Jacuzzi together, they seemed to be doing a lot more than just relaxing. The Jacuzzi was a little out of the way, but not *that* out of the way. She watched a bit, as she could, without obviously watching, and wondered what it would be like to be that unconcerned, that you could just catch some action at the workplace, and if people spotted you, it was their problem to decide whether to look away or observe.

That night she had a fleeting dream that she was the exercise instructor who was having sex in the hot tub. She felt proud of her body and simply happy to be slipping around with the man as the bubbles and froth swept around them. She was aware that people were watching and whispering, but this was just part of the atmosphere. Her bathing suit slipped off and swirled around on the surface of the water like a brightly colored flag while their slick bodies moved rhythmically around in the water.

This scene has water, bubbles, and warmth in a cocoon of sensuality that invites playful eroticism. Yet like some many exhibition dreams, it is a cocoon that is somewhat on display.

Even though this dream was triggered by an earlier event, it still has relevant implications for the dreamer. Any time the dreaming mind creates the experience of being someone else for you, pay close attention. Often all that keeps us from greater freedom or happiness is the idea of who we think we are. I'm not suggesting that you throw your identity away; but typically the *identified self* in our minds is much smaller and narrower than the totality of who we are. It is the difference between the functional you and the actual you. One of the reasons we admire certain people is because we recognize in them an aspect of ourselves that we probably don't identify with.

In this exhibition dream the couple seems proud of themselves and feeling somewhat naughty, but really they are just enjoying themselves and feeling *okay* with all the things that most of us are pretty careful with. They aren't worried about privacy; they aren't worried about their bodies or how they look. They aren't worried about their relationship or lack of it, nor about partners old or new. They are so free, enjoying sex in the hot tub the same way they enjoyed their workouts beforehand. In some respect, the relaxed quality of this dream is part of what makes it sensual and lighthearted.

In a sense, this dream suggests the sensuality of not keeping score, not grading performance, and not having every action attached to some greater implication. It is a relief, particularly to people who have highly organized lives subject to constant evaluation.

Dream Key #7

Introversion and Extroversion

I have a theory that extroverts are more comfortable with and intrigued by exhibitionism than are introverts. If you don't know whether you are an introvert or an extrovert, you're probably an extrovert. But you should know this very basic fact about yourself, because it will make life choices, relationships, and socializing infinitely more enjoyable if you do.

Essentially extroverts derive their rest and energy renewal by being with people. Introverts restore their batteries by stepping back and finding quiet and solitude. This basic difference may be more critical and influential on our choices even than whether we are male or female, gay or straight.

It also seems that our dreams and fantasies of exhibitionism say something about our desire for confidence in ourselves as sexual beings, our need for acceptance in the world. In these dreams we not only are admired and recognized, but by switching to the sexual channel, so to speak, we trigger a shift in others, too. Take a look at the following ideas and see if any of them apply to you.

Do you connect and converse better one-on-one, or in a group setting? If you find it more relaxing and *real* to be in a group, then you are probably on the extroverted side of the continuum. If you tend to save up your personality and spend it in quiet settings where you don't have to compete to be heard, then you may be more introverted.

What this implies in terms of your sex life is that you may feel more relaxed and accessible when you have absorbed the type of situation that restores your energy. Extroverts like to have sex after a nice party; they are in their best selves, jovial and sensuous, brimming with energy to exchange and burn.

Introverts are depleted after a party. They may start to feel edgy and raw, starved for solitude so they can process the party and get their energy and identity back. Introverts often have an unconscious toggle switch; they dissociate and minimize their presence when forced to "get through" an event or a series of events. If you could run a scanner over them to measure how alive they are, and how in their bodies they are, you would find they are pretty much not there! If you are an introvert, you know that sex when you are not at home in your body is a waste of time. Yes, sometimes it can pull you back in and ground you, but really, honestly, it's often another "event" to survive until you can finally have that restorative alone time.

This difference can be important to understand, particularly in a partnership, because the two types often pair up. So the extrovert is feeling sexy at times the introvert is feeling drained and not at home. The introvert feels sexy and full of imagination after a day at the museum or the library. The

extrovert is so bored and run-down from the lack of stimula-
tion, he or she needs some noise and action before they feel
happy again. After a scorching session of sex on Friday night,
the extrovert wants to meet for brunch on Saturday to do it all
over again. The introvert is fantasizing about meeting again
sometime next week. Both might rate the sex and the relationship as a "10," but their constitutions and energy cause them
to thrive in very different ways.

It's a tricky dance, but because these differences have everything to do with physical vitality as well as personality, the
more you understand about these distinctions, the richer intimacy can be.

CHAPTER EIGHT

The Anatomy Academy

Erotic dreams take great liberty with the human form, some-times providing no partner, but a very friendly free-floating penis that plays hide-and-seek. In other dreams you have the perfect lover, the perfect companion, and the perfect sex, but the guy just doesn't have a face!

For whatever reason, the body is the symbol of choice in dreams, and the tendency to make all things physical is a pow-erful component in dream symbolism. Dreams that involve and focus upon body parts are quite common, and though the story lines may differ, it is worth exploring the potential mes-sages in these brief, but memorable scenes.

The Problem with Ivy

One woman dreamed of going out in the woods for a romantic tryst, but partway there, she found something holding her back. As she looked down, she saw she had leaves of some kind growing out of the back of her ankles, and these were getting entangled in the brush along the pathway. She crouched down, and upon closer inspection saw that she had ivy vines growing from her ankles. She pulled on them, and though this didn't hurt, the vines wouldn't budge. Her partner was impatient and wanted to go on, and he pulled on her hand. She stood up but couldn't really walk anymore; her bizarre ivy growths were snarling everything up with each step she took.

Our feet and ankles symbolically represent our foundation in life: our early family life, and the worldview and emotional profile we formed in early years. When a dream shows a foreign object in a part of the body, as if "growing" there, it implies the presence of some cluster of emotions or behaviors that is outside our normal awareness. Vines sometimes symbolize patterns of belief or feeling that grow rapidly and become tangled and complicated. Interestingly, this cluster of confusion and sticky feelings was growing from her dream ankles, suggesting that this was her "Achilles' heel," or her weak spot. It also suggested that this tangle of feelings and relationship rules was probably not native to her individual nature, but something she had absorbed from early life.

The dreamer said that she came from the perspective of being cautious and detail-oriented, while her partner was impulsive and a risk taker. She loved being with him, but she sometimes felt encumbered by the numerous expectations and rules she had about everything that had to be planned and put in place before they could afford to be spontaneous. His daredevil ways excited her, but they also pushed her buttons and made her feel more compulsive about being careful and precise. The combination caused friction and confusion between them. Dreams have a wonderful way of taking complicated, unconscious patterns and illustrating them with vivid imagery. This couple is currently still working on making their dramatically different styles a strength instead of an impediment.

Why I Love My Bicycle Pump

One woman had a prolonged dream scene about a hazy figure who was climbing into her bed. She welcomed him, and they began to have sex, but stopped when she just couldn't feel much. He withdrew and she said, "Aha! *There's* the problem." She felt his erection was a little iffy, so she took the pump she used for her bicycle tires and sort of inflated it for him. They began again. This was much better, but rather quickly they were back at square one, and she could hardly feel anything going on. By this time she was getting frustrated and really wanted some vigorous thrusting or else. She again used the bicycle pump, not only to inflate his erection, but also just to make the whole anatomical situation super-sized. That seemed to do the trick. They had a nice time, and she vowed to always sleep with her bicycle pump on her nightstand.

In this scene the man was just a phantom fellow, with no identity or facial features. He was vaporish from the neck up, anatomically specific from the waist down. This was a dream between relationships, so likely the frustration she experienced in the dream was an expression of how she was feeling in general. Although men are most often associated with dreams of isolated body parts, women have these dreams, too. Sometimes systemically, we want sex without wanting to sort through the complexity of the relationship issues.

Perhaps I Should Have Told You . . .

A number of women report having occasional dreams in which they have both male and female genitalia. Often the surprise genitals are noticed when visiting the restroom, but sometimes the issue presents during dream sex.

One woman who was somewhat adventurous had a dream that she had picked up a cute guy and had brought him home for sex. They had been kissing and laughing as they walked home, and as soon as they stepped inside they started fumbling to get their clothes off, rolling around on the bed panting and making aren't-you-gorgeous sounds.

But by the time they got their clothes off, they both froze. Instead of the normal configuration of body parts, the woman now had a vagina and a penis. The penis had a jumbo erection that was poking out at her surprised date. Uh-oh. She had a moment of thinking: "Oh yeah, *right*, I forgot about that. I probably should have mentioned something." She was only feeling vague social embarrassment until she looked up at her date and saw him staring at her as if she were something from *Jurassic Park*. "He doesn't like the hard-on," she thought. So she tried to shove it sideways between her legs to conceal it.

Maybe they could work this out. But every time she moved or tried to embrace her still-stricken partner, her erection popped out like a banner.

In the symbolism of dreams, masculine anatomy sometimes represents masculine or out-in-the-world energy. This is certainly not absolute, but there are times when the dreaming mind makes this association. Feminine symbolism, including female anatomy can represent intuitive and feminine energy. Most theorists who work with dreams and with psychology assure us that we all have some of all these potentials; they rise to the surface during different times in our lives, and are responsive to different situations and needs. This dreamer is a person with dual energy, she is both masculine and feminine in strong doses, and it is possible that her dream was reflecting this high-voltage personality and essence. Although we envy people who have more energy and juice than the rest of us, they often find it hard to find a partner who can keep up with them, understand them, or who won't keep trying to tone them down. She did, from time to time, try to keep her companions comfortable by dimming her wattage a bit, so that she could have sex with them. Here she literally tries to hide her masculine power between her legs so that her partner will perhaps recover. As you probably might guess, this is also the dream of a fairly young woman, who is eager to have things go well, and thinks nothing of shoving aspects of herself into nooks and crannies if that is what it takes for the party to continue.

While some anatomical arrangements can tell us about ourselves symbolically, they can also give us glimpses into what it might be like to be someone else, with a different set of needs or different wiring.

Learning to Jerk Off

Several years ago I had a dream that I was standing out on the lawn in front of the home of a woman I liked. It was dark, and I was standing under a tree, staring up at the light in her bedroom window. I felt overwhelmed with desire, and unzipped my fly and took out my penis. Right away this got my attention. "I'm a *guy*," I thought. And oh, did it feel good to handle my penis. "No *wonder* men always want someone to handle these things," I thought. "This is *wonderful*." I began jerking off, feeling I had made a revolutionary discovery. At the same time, I had pretty much figured out that I was dreaming, that I was a woman dreaming of being a man, but it did nothing to diminish the fun I was having, or the significance of my discovery.

At the time of this dream, I was involved with a very "manly man" who was so different from me that it was hard for us to find a place where our interests and temperaments overlapped. I think the dream was trying to give me a different perspective, just a sample of what it is like to be in such a different body, capable of such different responses and feelings. One of the invaluable gifts of dreams is this magic of simulation, where an imaginary experience can provide lessons and memories that save time and transcend differences.

One of the things that makes dreams intriguing and perplexing is the way that the tone suddenly shifts when something unusual happens. This can sometimes hint that something "extra" is going on in a seemingly normal situation in waking life as well.

Put That Away, Mr. President

A divorced woman was struggling to keep custody of her son while her ex-husband was apparently gaining the upper hand.

One night she dreamed that she was negotiating a deal with then-President Clinton. She was trying to convince him of her perspective, and he was alternately arguing and flirting with her. She was getting desperate, on the verge of losing her temper, when she realized that somehow during their conversation, he had unfastened his pants and was showing her his erection. She was too startled to have much of a reaction, other than to stand up. He stood up too, grinning at her, as if this were all part of the game. She wasn't sure of the protocol here; it didn't seem right to say, "Put that away, Mr. President." At that point, she woke up.

It was not clear to her at first what this represented, until we began talking about power, authority, and sex. Then she quickly made the connection between her ex-husband and her dream. Her ex was, in a way, waving his power in her face, at the same time she felt that beneath it all, he wanted to strike out at her and also to keep her connected to him. There was a strange pulsation of desire that seemed to move through everything he did toward her. She had her hands full with the legal battle and trying to keep the climate from swamping her son. She hardly had time to analyze the subtle nuances she sometimes picked up around her ex's behavior. But her dreaming mind made note of the undercurrents in the situation, and took the time to create a little scene that posed the question: *Don't you think this is a little odd?* As it happened, her son did go to live with his father for a while, but it was more like a brief experiment that ran aground. To her delight, the husband soon tired of the situation, and her son was equally glad to move back home again.

Dream Key #8

Scoring the Anatomical Survey

Dreams have three ways of highlighting a body part. First, the body part may be free floating, or relatively solitary. Second, the body part may show up somewhere it isn't supposed to be. Third, the dream can highlight the part, providing a clue as to what is going on in waking life, like the woman with the ivy in her heels. When this happens, you can certainly consider what the body part may represent symbolically as a shortcut to interpreting the dream, and seeing if it has any gifts for you. Here are a list of body parts and the symbolism associated with them. This is a shortcut, a dream key, not the last word. Use it as a resource from which to make your own more personal connections.

Breasts/feminine
Penis/masculine
Feet/foundation, movement
Hands/autonomy, manifestation
Knees/flexibility, needs
Thighs/sexuality
Anus/perfectionism
Oral/communication, expression

Arms/strength
Shoulders/stoicism, responsibility
Ankles/history
Fingers/identity, creative expression
Thumb/will
Mouth/acceptance of nourishment
Teeth/personal power, choice
Throat/voice/acceptance

CHAPTER NINE

Sex with Friends

It's kind of embarrassing to have an erotic dream encounter with someone who is just a friend. There are lots of people you may like a great deal, but they don't really register on your sexual radar. Yet, sometimes, in your dreams, it's a different story. Why *is* that?

Sometimes, obviously, a friendship that is neutral and longstanding just takes a turn. In other instances, friends represent professional interests, or qualities we just want to try out in a partner. In some cases, dreams can give us an erotic assessment of the potential chemistry with another.

One woman had a dream from out of nowhere that she and a married coworker were rolling around having sex. In the dream she stopped by his desk and noticed that his sleeves were rolled up. She commented on his hairy arms, and they got into a flirtatious argument about what body hair implied about virility. He insisted that hairiness equated with staying power; she argued that was just an urban myth. She reached out to touch his arm, and they both felt a kind of heat rise between them. She straddled his chair facing him as they kissed. His erection pushed at her impressively, and soon they were on the floor breaking in the new carpeting. They had a nice time, and at least in the dream, his pro-hair argument seemed to have been validated.

In their real-life relationship the two argued all the time, but in a very friendly way that helped to pass the time. They were buds, having known each other for years. So she thought nothing of telling him about the dream she'd had. She thought he would get a kick out of it.

Instead, of course, he thought the anecdote was a signal, and perhaps in a way it was. He managed to get together with her in an alcove and kissed her out of curiosity to see if they had any chemistry. They did. After years of being family friends and work allies, they embarked on an affair that caught them both by surprise, especially when they couldn't stop. Their respective significant others found out, threatened them, demanded they end it, and they still couldn't stop. Eventually when it came right down to him losing his family, they both pulled back. But it was a *mess*.

This was a case, apparently, of her psyche registering some compatibility that she only perceived unconsciously. Perhaps it wasn't such a good idea to tell him about the dream. In the normal course of daily events, it is a slightly bizarre thing to share, and the door is wide open for it to be misconstrued. After the affair ended, he jumped through all the counseling hoops his (understandably) furious wife demanded, and they seemingly got through it. The woman is more aware that her dreaming mind may be astute at picking out potentially sexy partners for her, but has sworn off sharing them in casual conversation.

The Two-Dimensional Guy

Dreams intuitively scan potential situations for us all the time, including people we might become involved with.

One woman was conducting a flirtation with a man with whom she had little in common, but the vibes were there. She had the feeling he was going to ask her out soon, because the sexual energy was swirling around between them. She sensed he would be a good lover, but wondered how she could endure the things he liked; they were *so* boring. Also, they had been friends quite a while, and if they crossed this bridge, she didn't think it would work out. Then she would have mucked up a good friendship, and they would always be awkward together.

One night after seeing him and getting tingly, she had a dream that he took her out on his sailboat to finally consummate their mutual heat. Never mind that she didn't like water and didn't like boats; she thought she'd give it a go. The night sky was beautiful, and the sailboat was big. But as they loosened the necessary clothing, and he positioned her, she suddenly slipped down and over the side of the boat. He caught her in time, and she didn't fall in the water. He was pretty strong and hauled her back up. Once they got over that little shock, they tried again. This time he had thoughtfully tied a rope around her waist to be on the safe side. They rubbed their bodies together, and she reveled in how strong he seemed. She couldn't wait to feel him. But then, for no reason at all, she slipped again and went hurling off the boat toward the water. She was jerked, but not hurt by the rope, and he hauled her up again. This was getting ridiculous.

He suggested they should climb partway up the mast so he could gently tie her to the mast. They could have sex up there; it would be memorable. She looked up. She didn't like heights either, but they had to do something. They climbed the mast, and he tried to tie her to it, but she kept swinging out away from it alarmingly, like someone doing a bad impression of Tarzan. As she swung by and he missed her, she caught a glimpse of the boat from a different perspective as if from a distance.

Instantly she knew what the problem was. This scene was two-dimensional. They were in a picture. This was a picture of a boat on water, and she was a three-dimensional being trying to get in the picture, but sliding off it, because she was not flat enough to stick inside it. They would never be able to have sex, because she would just keep sliding out of the landscape of this picture of his life.

In the real world this man was not shallow or stupid; she liked him very much. But the dream was cautioning her that the differences she already sensed and worried about were even more profound, more essential than she realized. It was more than just a matter of enduring a few boring activities, they would not be able to fit no matter what they tried. Rather than go through a disappointment, she decided to steer clear of the opportunity to "try things out" with this man. And she believes she made the right decision.

The dreaming mind often sorts through possible partners

and opportunities. Just reflecting on their take on things can be useful, because of course your dreams come from your own mind and no one is more familiar with what you really need.

Dreams of sex with friends are not always about scoping out the possibilities, however. Sometimes the friends are symbolic and have an entirely different meaning.

The Radiant Resource

One woman periodically has a young friend come over and help with minor repairs and projects around the house. This man is one of those people everyone likes and trusts; he is a popular freelancer among her circle of friends. He is attractive enough, but not someone she would ordinarily look upon as a potential, or even a fantasy, sexual partner.

One night, though, she dreamed that the two of them were alone together. They lay down next to each other, smiling affectionately and delicately smoothing their hands over each other's bodies. At that point they were interrupted, and the woman had to attend to the myriad details of her busy life. They had been moving in a sexual direction when the action was interrupted, but there was also a compelling quality of quiet, stillness, and comfort with each other's presence that was just as memorable to her.

When she described the qualities of this friend, she said he was trustworthy, lovable, and radiantly positive. He is the kind of person that everyone instinctively loves and trusts, and feels uplifted in his presence.

The more she spoke, the more I felt she was describing her own qualities, for she is strikingly wise and gentle with an almost ethereal centeredness. When she is in a room, there seems to be a light coming from wherever she is sitting, as if she glows somehow, or there is an angel standing behind her. As we explored the possibility that this radiant young man was actually her radiance, she agreed that the dream was probably about her lack of time these days. She has little time to be "in the presence" of her spiritual and other interests in the way she craves. The interrupted love scene was a metaphor for her interrupted life these days. In this case the scene was not so much about literal sex as it was about union with the qualities she loves most in life and in herself.

Sometimes our dreams are pinpointing qualities we would like to have more of in a current relationship. Women often report dreaming of their lover's best friend or brother. They also sometimes borrow their girlfriend's husband in a dream.

The Borrowed Husband

A woman who is happily married reported that she frequently dreams of having sex with her girlfriend's husband. Her own husband is sensitive and just her style. Her friend's husband is a little rougher around the edges, and though he's a good guy, he's not someone she would have picked for herself even in her single days.

In the dreams she is usually in bed with her friend's husband, and they are making the most of some stolen time together. She feels badly about her husband, and her friend, but not badly enough to stop what she's doing. Besides, something about the taboo she is breaking makes it sexier.

This guy always falls on her like he's been away in prison

and hasn't seen a woman in years. He groans when he sees her body, and he travels all over her with his mouth and hands as if he wants to devour her. If the topic of their respective spouses comes up, he always reminds her that they just will never tell them about this, so no one will ever be hurt. This strikes her as idiotic and wrong, but somehow it makes her more aroused. In these dreams the fellow has apparently been fantasizing about her for years. He spends a long time showing her what he has been wanting to do with which parts of her body.

While her marriage is happy and strong, she does wish sometimes that her husband would be a little more carried away with things, a little more eager for her. Things are very civilized between them, as they both like it, but there are times when it would be lovely if things were a little more basic. She truly does not want her friend's husband, but it would be nice if she could inject some serum from him into her husband.

It appears these dreams give her the opportunity of experiencing a quality of intimacy she would like to have more of in her life without endangering her happy home or her friendship.

When we have serial or recurring dreams about a partner who is not a fantasy sexual figure, there is often another reason for the dreams. The dreaming mind may encourage you to move in a certain direction by depicting happy results from a union with someone who represents an occupation, a talent, or a pivotal decision.

The Eager Entrepreneur

One woman always wanted to go into business for herself, but had been advised it was better to work for a secure company. When she completed her education, she went to work for a large company that mass-produced craft items on a large scale. She enjoyed the work, but never lost the feeling that she would prefer to have her own business.

Years later she has intermittent dreams about a man she used to work with at that company. In the dreams they are getting back together after being out of touch and are realizing they have strong feelings for each other. He takes her to his studio, where he creates his own designs, and they have sex on the couch, the floor, or even on a tarp he has thrown down.

This is a man who left the company where they once worked to start his own business. She has not kept in touch with him and, in the ordinary course of life, never even gives him a thought. Yet he is clearly a powerful character in her dreams, evoking desire and affection, as well as *recognition*. She suspects, probably correctly, that he is an image for her longing to have her own business. When she thinks of him, she remembers him as "the guy who broke away and started a company of his own." Perhaps her dreaming mind is encouraging her to take a closer look at her hunger to run her own show. The dreams are set in his studio, rather than anywhere else in the world she might choose for fantasy sex, so this is likely significant as well. The studio is the place where this man is independent and creates designs. This is where she experiences excitement, fulfillment, and recognition; where she connects with her passion.

As important as sexuality and relationship are to women, there are also deep currents of passion for creativity, success, contribution, and expression in all of us. In days gone by, people spoke of having "a calling" for a certain activity or type of work. Modern life often does not invite the pursuit of subjective "callings," since most people have to be very strategic and tough-minded to chart their course. But your calling or special passion is still alive inside you. In some cases, dream partners who are "just friends," or not your style, have more to do with talents and timing than with your erotic taste.

There seem to be windows of opportunity in our lives, when we have the best chance to pursue something that has been unavailable to us for years. If you have a set of recurring dreams within a discrete period of time, it may be because the timing is right to take a fresh look at something you'd given up on. While it doesn't make sense to be foolhardy with your economic security, there may be a way for you to explore a unique expression of passion without sabotaging or sacrificing what you have. Remember, the conscious mind tends to be stuck with two choices all the time. It's all or nothing, no matter what the subject is. But the dreaming mind is connected with your creativity, intuition, and innovation. If some gift you have is rattling its cage to get out by triggering passionate scenes in your dreams, this may be the right time to give the idea serious attention.

Dream Key #9

What Those Friendly Lovers Can Teach Us

When a dream lover makes no sense due to lack of attraction or because he is just out of left field, you can get a handle on the meaning of his guest appearance by looking at them from a different angle.

1. Besides what you think of this person as a possible sexual partner, what quality would you use to describe him? Think occupation, personality, pivotal decisions, or temperament.

2. Is there anything in the location of the dream that suggests something to you? The art studio smacks of creativity, an auditorium implies a public forum, a laboratory implies research or investigation.

3. How sexy was the sex? In some dreams the sensations are so real that you wake up with vivid memories and may even feel a little out of it the next day. In other dreams there is a hazy sense that you have a tumble with someone, or fall in love, but the details are more a given assumption than a detailed sensory memory. If you simply recall that you were "with" a certain person, it is more likely that the dream is symbolic of union rather than necessarily about your sex life or preferences. There are exceptions to this assumption, but it is one way to start assessing your dream.

4. Notice the frequency of your erotic dreams. Frequent sexual dreams tend to have more to do with sex and less to do with intrapsychic messages or life choices.

5. If you believe your dreams might be providing clues about improving your relationship or your sex life, make a few notes about what those improvements might be. Sometimes there are positions, activities, or moods that have new appeal once you try them out in a dream. Always be careful in sharing erotic dreams with partners or friends and consider how others might receive your story.

PART THREE

Problems and Puzzlers

CHAPTER TEN

Personal Imbalance

The processes of dreaming can be biased toward your happiness. There appears to be a constant sifting of our experiences to mark what is fulfilling and what makes us feel stuck. Your current needs are fleshed out in dreams. Past memories or fantastic stories are used to get a handle on what to avoid and what to embrace in your life.

This doesn't imply that we should make all real-life choices try to match our dreams, but it is advantageous to review dreams for indicators of changing needs or increasing tension. Like a team of detectives tagging evidence of a crime, the dreaming mind is often ahead of the conscious mind in tallying up the signals of getting out of balance. Dreams of imbalance are often shocking, as they serve to put us on notice of patterns that are putting a kink in our well being. The important thing is to get an idea of what the dream implies and then to ask: How does knowing about this serve me?

The Boa Constrictor

Women's nightmares abound with elements that constrain, restrain, or shrink them. Whether it is a shrinking room or clothes too small, the psyche takes offense when factors in our lives reduce our freedom or authority.

One woman dreamed that after making love with her husband, she was just falling asleep. As she drifted off, she felt something moving in the bed. It pushed along up her thigh in an oozing progression, wrapped around her waist, then around her neck. This happened gradually. Before she knew it, she was encased by a huge white boa constrictor. Once she saw what it was, her heart pounded, but she couldn't move. She felt claustrophobic and paralyzed. It wasn't squeezing her to death, but it was much too tight, and she could barely breath. Her panicky struggles to take a deep breath finally woke her up.

This dreamer's marriage was largely positive and loving. But the setting in which she lived because of the relationship involved a tight and somewhat rigid community. She had converted to a new religion, moved to a new town, and lost her support system, all while adjusting to a new life. Underlying her myriad tensions, now that they were married and living in the highly structured setting, her husband, too, seemed to be somewhat more rigid, as if she were a reckless child who had to be prevented from folly. Sometimes it felt as if he were thwarting or squelching her for no reason other than some unwritten code. This was so subtle, she wasn't sure if she was imagining it, and was thinking negative thoughts because she was feeling tired and insecure.

The dream gave her an unmistakable heads-up that some factor in her life was indeed encasing her and causing her to feel she couldn't breath freely. Snakes can sometimes be phallic or sexual symbols. This constrictor in her bed, slithering along her thigh, certainly hinted that whatever was putting the squeeze on her was connected with her marriage.

A white boa constrictor seemed specialized and unique. When dreams shift the quality of an image, sometimes it is meaningful symbolically. She thought of her husband, his community, and her marriage as "good things." This made it even harder for her to process the sense of stricture she was experiencing. When you go off to live happily ever after, there is nowhere to really put the stress and sense of alienation from your old life. So what she felt engulfed by was a "white monster," something officially good that subjectively felt as if it was strangling her.

When we experience negativity around something that is officially a good thing, an amplification of tension occurs. Women often have a tendency to feel badly about their own anxiety in these circumstances. While our systems are trying to tell us something, we scold ourselves and judge our reactions. It is not clear where this pattern originates, but there seems to be something that causes us to feel ashamed when we are unhappy.

Imbalance sometimes occurs because we have taken the wrong path, but it also arises during transitions. Never avoid looking at a dream because you're afraid it will mean you have to leave. This dreamer was walking on eggshells to fit into her new world and was willy-nilly casting off her old ways to make this new life work. Every time there was a change, she simply discarded her needs or preferences to make up the difference. This is a crisis-management mode that is rather like making your portion of dinner smaller when unexpected company arrives. You get by with less. As a one-time solution there is nothing wrong with this. As a singular strategy for all occasions, it leads to a dead end because there's no *you* left.

As it turned out, this woman was happy with her marriage and ultimately happy with her new life. The dream was warning her of the gradual creeping strangulation that would happen if she chose to cope with change by erasing herself from the equation all the time. When a warning flag is waved in an anxiety dream, it is time to assess the situation, the future, and your options to counteract the imbalance. She felt she had to stop giving herself away and take steps to create a support system for herself in the new community.

When we deal with stress by a means that will ultimately come back to bite us, dreams often send a telegram warning of what lies ahead. The dream is usually far more dire than what we seem to be dealing with, yet the very drama can serve to let us know our feelings are real, and that the timing is good to move toward greater balance.

The Limbo Lover

One woman had a dream in which she was walking up the sidewalk and front steps to her lover's house. She was arched back, like someone in a limbo contest, leading with her pelvis and unable to really see where she was going. Since she knew the way, she hardly noticed this.

Her lover welcomed her, and they had sex on a bed that was suspended from the ceiling on long chains. This made a fun swinging motion as they moved, but she had to hold on to keep from falling off. They had great chemistry and, as usual, couldn't get enough of each other.

Initially she remembered this as a great sex dream, and it did reflect the chemistry and appetite they had for each other. But she wondered why she was bent so strangely. Physical alterations and distortions in dreams sometimes reflect imbalances. The physical image showed her bending over backward, leading with her crotch, and not seeing where she was going. She was involved in a fling and was hoping to turn it into a marriage, without really taking in the reality that the other party was not in the same place she was in terms of long-term goals and wanting a family. His bed was literally "swinging," rather than being attached to the ground.

Many of us have had a relationship or two that we entered as if by following a magnetized pelvis. When our goals are truly in another direction, our dreams may let us know that we're in a position that we really don't want to sustain permanently.

Stapled Mouth

One woman had a dream that she was having sex with her boyfriend with their usual intensity. She wanted to make some noise, the pleasure was so intense, but then she noticed that she couldn't get her mouth open. In the way of dreams, she could see herself, and her mouth had been stapled shut with building staples. This struck her as odd, but she was occupied with sex and paid little attention. There was no pain involved, just the striking image.

Then her dream flashed to other scenes, sitting around the Christmas tree, handing out packages. Nodding because she could neither speak nor smile because her mouth was sealed with staples. Making breakfast for her family, passing scrambled eggs to her kids, gesturing them to eat because her mouth was sealed.

This striking image made her a bit queasy because her boyfriend was a building contractor, and it was easy to see that somehow her ability to express herself was being sealed off in their relationship. She wanted to marry and have a family, but the dream's fast-forward into the future warned her that she wouldn't want to go through life with the real-life equivalent of this situation.

Sometimes there are unspoken deals or contracts in relationships, as there are in families. One person is playing the role of the smart one, one is playing the role of the dumb one, and the smart one will invariably correct whatever the dumb one says regardless of the merits of the conversation. In families, one sibling will be the good kid, another the rebel. One sister will be "the pretty one," and the other sister will sometimes treat her body badly or negate her own beauty, not because of anything "real," but because of her subjective identification as "not the pretty one." These patterns seldom occur to us consciously, but when they contribute to an imbalance or unhappiness, they may be dramatized in a dream.

This dreamer was not being told to shut up, nor would she have tolerated such treatment. But there *was* an undercurrent of criticism occurring, and it was having a cumulative effect.

To borrow a line from Perry Mason, if everything you say can and will be held against you, then you tend to say less and less.

One of the things that made this dream so compelling was the future preview of her with her not-yet-born family. Although she stayed with the relationship for a while, eventually the sacrifices seemed too great and they parted company. She now believes that a critical step in finding the right person is being able to walk away from the wrong person. We never want to part from those we care about or have grown used to, but sometimes our dreams nudge us to get on a more life-affirming path.

Shark-Infested Waters

A lovely and very sociable woman became involved with a sensitive, introverted man. They had a wonderful time in the initial phase of their relationship. His sensitivity made him an extraordinary lover who seemed to know everything that would drive her wild. It was as if he knew her body and her imagination better than she did. They also had long intense conversations, just the two of them, about all sort of topics. This was amazing to her. Here was a man who only wanted to have long conversations and long sessions of sex in which her body was like a temple at which he worshiped. This, a gal could get used to.

Her friends noticed she wasn't going out as much and didn't have time for them, but then this often happens when women fall in love. The woman was at first happy to snuggle at home with her new partner. She sometimes wished she could pry him out of the house, but he grew irritable when she forced the issue. Over the months that followed, she grew restless and pale. He seemed to be thriving in their cocoon, but she felt as if her lifeblood were being drained away. She wanted her friends, her group meetings, her hobbies and classes. The unwritten rule was: We don't go anywhere. As one of the most extroverted souls on the planet, she literally became sick as a result of being cut off from the things that fed her vitality.

One night she dreamed they were on a cruise together. Finally, she thought, she could socialize, dance, and mingle with the crowd. But he wanted to stay in their cabin. They made love, and she found herself wishing that for once he would stop interminably fondling every inch of her and just *do* it. She wanted more than anything to get out on deck and meet the other passengers.

When they did emerge finally, they found people gathering around and looking over the sides of the ship with concern. Everyone was talking about the fins they saw circling the bow: There had to be hundreds of sharks down there. On such a large ship they were not in any apparent danger, yet it lent a morbid tone to the cruise. The sharks were following the ship almost like vultures, as if they expected someone on board to die and fall overboard.

Shuddering, the woman and her boyfriend left the deck and went back downstairs to take their minds off the unsettling sight. Once downstairs, though, they heard people scuttling toward the engine room. There had been a body discovered down there. Curious, drawn against their will, they followed others who were going in the engine area to see. There, they found not one body, but stacks of corpses against the walls, as if people had been dying on this ship for a long time and the bodies were just being tossed into the engine compartment. Now they understood. Somehow the sharks had picked up the smell of decaying flesh on the ship, and they were circling hungrily.

This dream is exceptionally explicit in depicting the "love boat" this woman has been on as a "ship of death." While this was a melodramatic version of events, her health in waking life had been eroding to an alarming degree; the series of specialists she visited could not pinpoint what was wrong with her. She wasn't really dying, but when we feel our spirits are dying, the sensation is almost the same, and who can say to what extent our systems begin to unravel when we lose hope?

Sharks often symbolize troubles and fears. These sharks seemed to reflect her sense of being surrounded by a dark circle of antilife, something that wanted to consume her, but would not allow for her survival. The corpses under the deck seemed to reflect and dramatize her feeling of slowly dying. Whenever she contemplated the sensation that she was fading away, she would stuff that idea out of sight, almost the way the bodies had been tossed below.

Morbid dreams often explore situations in our lives that are "deadening." Extroverts not only prefer being social, they *need* to be around people. The introverted man in this relationship was not a monster. I suspect he truly loved this woman, who was as bright as a sun and must surely have lit up his home. As things evolved, her health problems precipitated the need for her to urgently reduce the stressors in her life, and with mutual regret the two parted. Not long afterward, the man found a "homebody," who was happy with his lifestyle, and they became engaged. The woman quickly recovered from her mysterious health maladies once she returned to the lifestyle and the rhythms that nourished her. She too is in a new relationship and is reportedly thriving.

This anecdote is not meant to imply that introverts and extroverts cannot be happy together. Often these two types revel in the differences and perspectives each can bring to a partnership. It seems critical that we learn how necessary it is for each type to have access to the circumstances that restore and "feed" them. You would not consider saying to a loved one: "All the things that make you feel alive and happy are now off limits. Instead you will spend the rest of your life being drained and frustrated with no hope of regaining your energy." Yet, by insisting that a partner of a very different type live exclusively in our universe, that is, in a sense, what we try to do.

Sometimes people share with me that their partner has everything "on their list," and is a great find, and they are lucky to have them. Yet they feel miserable, even depressed. Sometimes discontent is not about the person you are with, but about the lack of energy-restoring circumstances in your lifestyle.

Dream Key #10

Claiming the Gift in Warning
Dreams and Feelings

Transitions

Special pacing and nurturing are necessary when you are going through a transition. Even a truly positive transition can bring with it a sense of crisis. It's important to let yourself own the negativity of a "good thing," and to trust that you will make good decisions for yourself and your future even under pressure. You have the right to give yourself time to adjust and you have the right to cultivate and maintain a support system, whatever you are doing.

Short-term Versus Long-term

In the throes of the moment, we may not have much of a feeling for the future. But dreams and intuition start sending signals when we have taken a road that is not leading us to the future we truly want. If you are unsure about this, sometimes it's possible to set a time limit on a connection. Rather than drift too long, you might just mark your calendar six months ahead to revisit your decision and evaluate things then.

Negotiable—Nonnegotiable

There are always things we can compromise on that don't really reduce our quality of life or enjoyment of a connection. Some things, though, are deal-breakers and won't bear the test of time. Its useful to have some sense of clarity in your own mind about what is mandatory to your happiness and what is flexible.

One of the most sensual women I've ever met told me that when she met a man who was slightly less accustomed to adventurous intimacy, she flatly told him, "Look, I want to do these kinds of things and sex is very important to me. If you're not interested in having these kinds of experiences, then we aren't going to have a relationship." Apparently the man accepted this requirement without hesitation, because they not only stayed together, but are now grandparents. Word has it they are still shocking their friends because of the way they rock the cabin walls on group vacations.

Knowing what you truly want and genuinely need is not a guarantee of getting it, but it certainly improves the odds.

CHAPTER ELEVEN

Erotic Nightmares

Nightmares often surge when we've reached an impasse with a problem or pressure in our lives. Most of us soldier on with challenges for as long as possible, and when we hit the brick wall for the umpteenth time, we then feel overwhelmed. At this point of crisis or peak torment, nightmares usually start bubbling up. But psychic crisis is not an indication that a problem is insoluble, nor that the dreamer is having a break-down. Some nightmares are valuable expressions of the life force screaming in protest. If we can summon the willpower to explore them, we will not only feel better about ourselves and about our problems, but may well discover important clues about the resolution of the crisis, or at the very least some sense of how to position ourselves to weather the storm.

Maybe because sex and relationships are so important to us, women tend to have a fair number of erotic nightmares, in which sex and desire turn inside-out, becoming weapons of torture or unwelcome pursuit.

These dreams are paradoxical; no one wants to talk about them because they are shocking and disturbing. We wonder where such imagery comes from. Even so, people tend to feel a need for answers when a dream is frightening or contains horrific imagery.

Rape

Women seem to dream of rape in cycles. Fortunately the dreams do not appear to be precognitive shadows of crimes around the corner. For the most part, these dreams appear to use rape as a symbol for a revolting personal violation of another kind.

One woman who was trying to work her way up in a company was passed over for promotion. The opportunity went to someone less qualified but more high-gloss in a superficial sense. Not only that, but she learned she was to have a new male supervisor much younger than herself that she would begin reporting to. The whole episode felt like a defeat, and also an insidious victory by some subtle network of power that she didn't understand.

Around that time she had a dream that she went into the lavatory at work and was accosted by a young thug who forced her back into a stall and raped her. She fought back, but there was nothing she could do and she didn't want to be hurt even more if she could help it. Bruised and traumatized, she was left there by the rapist, who laughed at her on his way out the door.

This gritty nightmare reflected her sense of having been

hurt and violated by recent events. She poured her emotions and talents into the company, imagining that she was accruing value in the eyes of management and coworkers. Instead, it seemed she had been used and "taken." When we dream of rape, it is so horrible that we tend to forget other aspects of the dream. Because of this overwhelming horror, it can be useful to paraphrase the dream to get some distance from it, and see whether it may be a metaphor for some other type of wounding. If you look at this dream and substitute the words *used*, *abused*, and *violated* for raped, it begins to make sense. The fact that the scene took place at work, of course helps to make a connection as well. The dream could be described this way: *I am at work and am used, abused, and violated. Then I am laughed at*. With this short sentence, it becomes much easier to see what is going on.

Interpreting dreams like this one are helpful immediately in at least two ways. First, it helps to take some of the horror out of a remembered scene like this, when you know it is symbolic. She was reassured. Second, like the victim of a crime, she realized that it would take some time for her to recover from the "wound" she felt around the work situation. She needed to give herself some room to grieve over the loss of the mental picture she had previously had about the situation, before she reacted or responded to it with choices of her own.

Pursuit with a Weapon

Many women have dreams that involve being pursued by a man carrying a gun or a knife. He may be a serial killer or rapist, or he may be someone who just has it in for the dreamer. Usually it is a dark, unknown figure, who is always just outside in the darkness, watching and waiting for his chance. In the way of dreams, these women sense he wants to probably kill them, but also wants to get at them for his own dark purposes.

One girl dreamed that she was at her high school at night, having stayed there for a play rehearsal. She expected to catch a ride home with others in the play and ducked into the bathroom quickly before they headed out. When she emerged from the bathroom, the hallway was quiet, dark, and deserted. She realized they must have forgotten her and gone home without her. She walked down the dark hallway trying to decide whether to head for her locker, the parking lot, or the pay phone. Her footsteps sounded hollow, echoing in the empty building. She noticed then that what she had thought was an echo, was really another set of footsteps. She walked faster; the echoing footsteps sped up behind her. She rounded a corner and glanced over her shoulder. There was a dark figure carrying something. Some light reflected on a gleaming surface, and she saw it was the blade of a knife. She broke into a run and cut through a passage that was a short cut to outside. The footsteps ran behind her. As she ran and became more agitated, she finally awoke, still frightened.

She had this dream a few times, with several variations, but always with a man carrying a knife and always at her school. In the symbolism of dreams, guns and knives combine a number of elements, representing violence, threat, and power. In dreams with sexual undertones, these weapons tend to be carried by men, in pursuit of women, and they are brandished at the victims or carried in front of the men, straight out, like malevolent erections.

This young woman was experiencing some unwanted attention at school. Fortunately the real-life situation was not as threatening or as violent as the dream version. Because of the constraints and enmeshment of high school, this girl felt a bit trapped by the variables in her situation. Adolescence is a time of exquisite excitement at burgeoning sexual attractiveness and power. Being a sexual person is what you want to be at that age. When something dark and sticky seemed to attach itself to her because she was shining as bright as the sun, it was alarming. She may have felt even more stricken when something disturbing seemed to be thrown into the mix of what had previously been a source of satisfaction and delight. She decided to run the situation by her mother and her friends to get their suggestions and developed a plan to reduce her exposure to the unwanted attention.

Home Invasion or Burglary

A particularly common nightmare deals with someone trying to get into your home. Many women report variations on this theme, not all of them with sexual overtones. In many cases, dreamers race from window to window trying to secure their house because they can hear someone outside who is trying to get in. When these dreams have a sexual component, the intruder usually makes it inside, and unfortunately the dreamer is forced to negotiate or struggle with him.

These dreams generally have nothing to do with fantasy, and are instead signs of external pressures or internal struggles.

In one particularly violent dream, a woman tried to secure her home against an intruder and was able to lock every door in the house. She retreated to her bedroom to hide and call the police, then realized in horror that she had neglected to lock the sliding-glass door into her bedroom. The intruder walked in easily and stood in the middle of the room, watching her and smiling unpleasantly. She darted away toward the phone, but he quickly grabbed her and picked her up, tossing her on the bed like a doll. She bounced and scrambled up again, but he caught her and pushed her to the floor, straddling her and sitting on her. The breath was pushed out of her, and she looked around for anything that might be within reach to use against him. Her hand closed on something, a heavy jar of vitamins that was under the bed. With all her might she smashed the jar into the side of his head. Blood spewed around them, and he fell sideways off her. She had caved his head in, and she slid away toward the phone to call the police, so sick she couldn't look at the prone form of the intruder as she dialed for help.

This woman had experienced some rough relationships in earlier years, and although her life had regained equilibrium, occasionally she still felt "embattled" in her dreams. When dreams depict blood and gore, even when it comes from another character, this is usually associated with a sort of wounding that the dreamer herself has experienced.

This dream burglar trespasses in the bedroom, not another room in the house, and he is powerful enough to toss her about like a doll. However, the dreamer fights back with rare ferocity. In the discipline of dream analysis, when a dreamer takes action on her own behalf, it is called "agency." It simply means being an advocate for yourself and challenging your monsters even if you do not ultimately win. Possibly, in addition to feeling powerful and whole again, she has also been nourishing her spirit and taking care of herself in a variety of ways, because we see that when the demons try to sneak in and torment her, she fends them off with a symbol of deliberate self-care: vitamins.

Clearly, we all have struggles that we wrestle with for years, often for lifetimes. We can be dismayed to continue to dream of some trauma, years after it has happened. Yet when dreams show us fighting on our own behalf or taking some action to improve the nightmare, this is a strong clue that the process of recovery is underway.

Bigfoot and Company

A prevalent nightmare with sexual overtones deals with big hairy creatures chasing us through the woods. In some dreams these are anomalous creatures, like perverted Bigfoots. Dreamers describe them as a combination of bear, gorilla, and man.

Other dreamers always see a big bear in the forest, or a primate of some sort. Whatever they are, these creatures mean us no good, and dreams of this sort involve long-drawn-out scenes of racing through the woods, falling over tree roots, and running as fast as you can.

Often these dreams are recurring. They arise spasmodically through the years, and may seem to have no apparent connection to a real-life stressor. But if you step back from the image, these themes involve a big hairy monster that stands on two legs and is out to "get" you. Whatever the goal is, you certainly don't want it to catch you.

In many cases, these hairy predators are symbolic of the negative predatory side of sexuality. The hairy creatures are like caricatures of something powerful and hypersexual out to consume us.

Women have these chased-by-a-bear dreams when they are experiencing some negative "scent" of predation around them. These scenes are also more common to women who have been victimized or who were abused as youngsters. In some cases, these dreams can be used as a signal to recognize when something is making you uneasy. Instead of talking yourself out of your instincts, let the dreams help you to pay attention to the feeling that something feels creepy or off base.

Tortured by Tom Hanks

Just as it is hard to know what to do with negative feelings about positive transitions, it is also hard to know what to do with negative feelings about a positive person. In the weights and measures of the psyche, feelings that have no place to go become just as dramatic as feelings that come from a truly horrendous circumstance.

One woman had a series of dreams that she was married to the actor Tom Hanks. In these dreams they had been married for some time and had an officially good relationship. They had a very active sex life, and the dreams often began with their vigorous lovemaking. But then Tom would turn mean, saying cruel things to her and threatening her. In one dream he hauled her out of bed after sex and pushed her up against a wall. Then he started throwing darts and knives at her from across the room like one of those circus acts. The knives missed her flesh, but pinned her to the wall through her clothing.

In real life this woman had long been partnered with a man that she truly loved. They had a child together, and she had assumed they were partnered for life. But in the year during which she had these dreams, he had announced that he wanted to have an open relationship for a while, in which they would both see and sleep with other people. Although she could theoretically understand this in principle and went along with it, she felt betrayed and tormented by it. Somehow it felt as if the point of the change was not increased sexual freedom, but some passive-aggressive torture aimed at her. Eventually she decided to end the relationship because it simply felt that everything good was being eroded by their new lifestyle.

She described Tom Hanks as someone "everybody likes." Her partner was similar in that everyone thought he was the salt of the earth. She, too, felt he had many fine qualities, but as in the dreams, there was a streak that she found she couldn't embrace. She has since married a very different type of man and is more comfortable with their commitment and their relationship.

Dream Key #11

Decoding Erotic Nightmares

Nightmares usually appear in patches associated with a set of real-life pressures. Keep the questions below for reference if you or someone you know has a bad dream. Remember two important points: First, the worse the dream, the greater the potential benefit you will gain from looking at it. Second, the best way to reduce nightmares is to review them. Pushing them out of your mind generally makes them worse. Turn toward them, not away from them.

1. **Timing.** When did the nightmares start? Stress comes in time capsules. Like the woman who worked with her ex and dreamed of the snakes, you can trace the onset of your nightmares to the beginning of the real-life stressor that is triggering them.

2. **History.** If you've had this theme for years, it is more likely associated with a past experience or a dynamic put in place by your early experiences. This is the kind of dream you have once a year, but have always had.

3. **Theme.** Identify the quality of the horror. Is it violation, betrayal, menace, or disempowerment? The theme will help you identify what part of your life is exerting this pressure on you, and help you determine what to do about it.

4. **Short-term Tactic.** Like an accident victim who needs first aid, you need to do something right now to "stop the bleeding." Add people to your team by sharing the dream or your fears with them. Get expert help if you need it. Keep making phone calls until you get what you need. Take safety precautions if you need to, and hunker into whatever your survival mode is to shore up your energy.

5. **Long-term Strategy.** Not only should you do something to stop the bleeding, but you've also got to make a plan so that things will get better over the long haul. Maybe you can't execute this plan right away, but *make* it.

CHAPTER TWELVE

Infidelity

Infidelity dreams come in two flavors: either your partner cheats, or you do. Both genres involve impulsive actions and dire repercussions; it's difficult to know which type of dream is more unsettling. When a partner is unfaithful in a dream, there is often some triggering emotion that mushrooms into a theme of betrayal. But when dreamers find themselves cheating in dreams, the precipitating feelings are usually quite different. In the dreams that follow, the underlying currents will become clearer.

He's Cheating Already?

There seem to be two phases of relationships when we are most prone to dreams of spousal infidelity. The first is during the time of settling in with your partner or spouse, within the first few years. The second is years later, when things have become so comfortable and rumpled between you two that it sometimes seems your libidos got left in the laundry hamper.

Newly united couples should have a good three years of ideas and energy before they take a deep breath, so why do so many of us quickly begin to dream that our partners are going astray?

One woman said that shortly after she moved in with her fiancé, she began having odd dreams that he was cheating. In these dreams it turned out that he preferred an entirely different sort of woman; different in appearance, style, body type, and personality. Their relationship was some sort of an experiment, but what he really wanted was some other "model" of woman. In the dreams he had found an irresistible example of this preferred type, and he was going off to have compulsively riveting sex with her whenever he had the chance. In the dreams he seemed oblivious to her presence when she saw them together; he just went on humping the creature who was all tanned legs and long hair. She didn't know which made her feel worse, the betrayal or the knowledge that she wasn't what he wanted after all; she was the wrong type of woman.

In their real-life relationship everything was going well. They continued to enjoy each other physically, and their plans for the future were moving smoothly ahead. She had no sense of any real threat to their relationship. Yet as a relationship transforms from liaison to partnership, the stakes go up. This dreamer, like many, found that she became vulnerable to fears of losing what she had found in a way she had never felt before. Her life ahead was like treasure she was guarding, and though there were no realistic threats around, the very quality of declared permanence changed everything. It's like throwing your heart in the sand and saying: This is where I'll make my stand. It won't be okay if something spoils this one.

The dreaming mind considers love, relationships, and family as matters of life-and-death seriousness. It becomes a sentinel, scanning the horizon for any hint of trouble and producing warning dreams that amplify those threats. In this background of high stakes increased vulnerability and dream vigilance, shifts in the nuances of the relationship register like earth tremors beneath your feet. As couples grow close, warmth and intimacy increase. Yet there can also be a bit of worry about how it will work, whether you can be monogamous forever, and how it must be for your partner. There is also the feeling that you have bought the sedan instead of the sports car, and you can only hope that everything will work and be satisfactory.

For this dreamer there was the feeling that the sizzle that had been her passport to the relationship might be dimmed or misplaced over time. What if, as a steady diet, she wasn't what he wanted after all? Her nightmare, that there was some special "type," and she just wasn't it, reflected this irrational but very real fear.

Her fiancé seemed to be going through some kind of archetypal metamorphosis. He attacked his work with vigor and seemed feverish in his need to get their home and their life ahead ready. There are studies suggesting that expectant fathers go through a stage of working harder and longer, as if by instinct to help provide for the incipient family. It seems that most of us "gear up" for the new stages in our lives, and carving greater success is often part of it. At a time when the dreamer was unconsciously worrying whether she could continue to inspire passion in her partner, the partner was becoming obsessed with working longer hours, finishing home improvements, and building a life. Logically, this was all good. Unconsciously, it felt as if the spotlight of passion that used to shine on her was slowly turning elsewhere.

This sense of being left in the cold was irrational, but real. Fortunately, though, over time, she essentially outgrew the sensation, and the dreams stopped. There was no real-life unfaithfulness, and she no longer fears that she may somehow be the "wrong type of woman."

Striped-Hair Bimbo

The second phase when dreams of unfaithfulness arise usually comes after a relationship has been in place for some time. At this point things are comfortable and secure, and the dreams come like a sucker punch in the night, leaving us furious and suspicious in the morning.

One woman dreamed that her husband was lying next to her in their bed with a bimbo underneath him; she could see the woman's multicolored dyed hair spread out on the pillow. In the morning she awoke and sat up watching his sleeping form, struggling with the urge to smack him because the dream had seemed so real.

Yet in the real world, so far as it is possible to be sure, there seemed to be nothing going on. The only thing that drew the husband away was his addiction and commitment to his hobbies, notably fishing. We can never be sure if the brilliantly dyed hair of the dream bimbo was symbolizing a rainbow trout, but it is often the case that *anything* that leaves us feeling like second best can morph into "the other woman" in our dreams.

It is the emotion of betrayal and abandonment, of feeling like something other than first on the list, that seems to trigger these dreams. He isn't really doing somebody else, but he is passionate about something else, and that can stir up uneasiness. Sometimes there is some negotiating to be done; sometimes acceptance and reframing the enthusiasms of those we love can settle our rankling feelings.

Deal-Breakers

Just as the initial stage of commitment triggers nightmare scenarios of your partner cheating, this is also a time when women dream they impulsively have a little fling that ruins everything. Whenever we're up to something big and important in life, we are bound to have a few dreams about dropping the ball. The more you care about an event or transition, the more likely you are to dream ahead of time about disasters that wipe out your happiness.

In these dreams the women never *mean* to cheat. They temporarily lose their focus, that's all. They run into an old lover, and before they can fully explain about their newly committed state, their clothes are off and they honestly forget all about it. It's only after the lights come back on that they realize something is horribly wrong. Though they try to tell themselves to go for the next best thing to being faithful, that is—hiding this forever—it never works out. The fiancé, coming as a surprise, walks in, and there is a stormy breakup and the dreamer's life is ruined. She stands there, clothes pressed to her sweaty, teary body, and wonders how she could *ever* have been so careless.

One woman had versions of this dream when she got engaged to her future husband. She wasn't tempted to cheat on him and didn't envision being tempted in the future. But the dreams seemed to reek of fear that she would, through some thoughtless moment of distraction, destroy her happiness. In her dreams she had sex with airline pilots and truck drivers, old boyfriends and coworkers. Each time her fiancé appeared and was devastated and unforgiving in the face of her betrayal.

As their relationship evolved, the dreams stopped. They were, in a sense, a sort of performance anxiety about marriage, relationship, and her life ahead. It was as if she kept worrying: What if I mess this up? One of the only ways she could destroy the relationship would have been by being unfaithful. Though it certainly wasn't likely in waking life, in her dreams she was as impulsive as an actress in an X-rated movie. In her past, she had found herself in a few relationships and a few beds that were somewhat unintentional at the outset. Her dreams seemed to be working through some fear that she might "accidentally" mess up this high-stakes game of happiness. She didn't. But the more significant the threshold we're about to cross, the more likely we are to dream about sabotaging it somehow or having it taken away from us.

Separation Anxiety

One woman had a theory that you should never be separated from your spouse for more than a couple of weeks, because if you are, one or both of you will be unfaithful.

When she and her spouse were about to be separated for about a year, she had many anxiety dreams about the upcoming separation. The anxiety manifested in the form of dreams in which she could not control herself and was repeatedly unfaithful in her husband's absence. In the dreams she became involved with a family friend and with a coworker, as well as with fictional characters who did not really exist. In each dream not only did she feel she let her marriage down, but her husband also found out somehow and demanded a divorce.

The dreams were loud protests against the upcoming separation, and the scenes played out her fears that somehow this would ruin her marriage. The dreams also seemed to go to great lengths to show her as a loose cannon, a woman who had no control and who could not keep her life or herself on track. Certainly the circumstances forcing the separation, though agreed to as necessary, felt like they had taken control out of her hands. She felt like a bundle of emotions, urges, and instincts twitching in protest but unable to do anything.

Underlying these dreams may have been the belief that the woman "keeps things together," and that it was up to her not only to survive the separation, but also to make sure the marriage and the future survived the separation. This was a lot on her shoulders, and it exacerbated her fears that she might somehow not be up to the challenge. This chapter in her life was years ago. She survived, and was apparently not triggered into nymphomania by the absence of her spouse. The reality of their separation was challenging, but not nearly as horrible or "deadly" as her dreams.

In observing performance and transition anxiety in dreams, there is a tendency for people who are very capable and reliable to have powerful anxiety dreams of doing things wrong, forgetting to show up, or not being prepared. The more competent and careful the individual, the more likely they are to have these types of dreams. It may be that these scenes are like an anxiety-defrag that the brain performs to try and keep everything working smoothly. Or that for these people, not living up to their responsibility is the ultimate nightmare, and so this is what they dream when they experience pressure.

We can learn from infidelity dreams that, in most cases at least, literal unfaithfulness does not appear to coincide with them. We can also realize that the early stage of a committed relationship is where the stakes go up and consequently where we may ruminate in our dreams on possible disasters. We women take special pleasure in being the object of our lover's passions, and any shift that moves the heat of that spotlight away from us feels *wrong* and potentially threatening, at least until we settle in.

We are just as afraid of being unfaithful, at least in that early stage, as we are of our lovers being unfaithful.

Later in the relationship, when both parties are comfortable and exploring other interests, we may have dreams of a spouse being unfaithful. Usually there is some factor that is occupying his time and energy, whether it is volunteering, overtime, or hobbies.

Separations can induce a lot of anxiety, provoking dreams of infidelity in which one or the other partner ruins everything. These dreams remind us that our relationships are fluid, living things, with rhythms that shift. We have seasons of feeling close and sensual, other seasons when we feel less sure of things and less content. Part of weathering these seasons is knowing the signs of tension in yourself and in your dreams, and knowing these scenes for the anxiety dreams they are.

Dream Key #12

What Is Really Going On?

1. If you do the cheating in your dreams, ask yourself whether you're really having "performance anxiety" dreams. If so, you will likely also be having dreams about forgetting things, wedding disasters, and public embarrassment. Important transitions call for desperate measures, and you will want to take special care of yourself now. This is not the time to be distant from girlfriends because you are short on time. Make time; you need to debrief and get some fresh air.

2. If your spouse is the dirty rotten scoundrel, make a list of the things that you feel are pulling him away from you. This isn't to get you mad at him; this is to give you something to review and try on to see what you think is going on. If your instinct tells you there's no real-life infidelity, then trust your instinct. Remember, the deeper mind doesn't want to feel that drifting-away feeling; it's a big deal. Knowing how this works can help you keep your equilibrium and focus on ways of feeling close that will please both of you without being clingy.

3. Consider the stage of the relationship. Is this the newly committed anxiety stirring, or is this taken-for-granted resentment producing a blame movie? If you're with

someone who has a passionate hobby, you've got to let them have it. Lots of couples make deals about this, negotiating and trading time and permissions with each other. Do what works for you and ask your friends for their stories. Remember, the infidelity in your dreams is only a symbolic deal-breaker; in real life this is going to work out.

CHAPTER THIRTEEN

Nowhere to Make Love

Some dreams are like prolonged adolescent nightmares where you and your sweetie get together, but can't find anywhere to be alone. There's no place, no room, no car, no woods; everywhere you go someone or some thing makes it a no-go. The factors that ruin our dream episodes often represent real issues that short-circuit our love lives. These dreams, while annoying, can be very worthy of our attention because their exaggerations can make the nature of our challenges much more clear.

From Here to Eternity

One woman had taken a breather from her relationship when the problems she'd had with her partner seemed insurmountable. Although it was difficult and painful, she also felt relieved at the absence of friction. Part of her wanted to just run back to him, and part of her was refreshed by the peace she felt. It was hard to know if they were doing the right thing by separating.

She had a dream that she and her lover had somehow gotten back together and had decided they were meant to be together. They met on a beach and ran to each other, kissing and then sliding into the sand together, rolling around with abandon as the water splashed up onto them. Unfortunately, she seemed to be lying on some kind of sea creature, perhaps a jellyfish, which kept poking her and stinging her in the back. Her partner still wanted to have sex, but she really could hardly catch her breath the stings hurt so much. It was like someone was sticking a hard, bony finger into her kidneys. She wriggled away and stood up. Her partner rose up to help her, and they staggered off to find a better location.

This scene is typical of the aborted-sex themes that seem to highlight the lack of a good place to have sex. This woman's mind was apparently trying to clarify to her that although she now missed her partner and missed having sex, there were real issues, real pain involved that needed to be examined with delicacy and time. To rush back with Hollywood drama might only be asking for surprising pain.

Hiding the Evidence

One woman who was getting serious about her partner was hoping they might become engaged soon. Everything was going well, except that he seemed unusually jealous of her, and of her past. Still, they came from different worlds, and in his world things were orderly. It was one of the things she liked about him. As they grew closer, she began to learn that speaking of her past was not a good idea and referring to her many male friends was also not recommended. She developed a habit that became second nature, to keep her casual anything-goes side under wraps when she was with him.

She dreamed that through some snafu, she had killed somebody. It looked like the body was male, although she couldn't quite place him. She was worried because she knew her boyfriend was coming by soon, and this wasn't the sort of thing he would understand. She had to hide the body somewhere so he wouldn't see it. She pulled the corpse by its feet down the basement stairs, the head thumping distressingly on each step. She tried not to think about it; all would be well if she could just cover it up with something. She would deal with it later. She covered it up with some old blankets that were down there.

By now she was sweating and shaking, but still gearing up to meet her boyfriend. She sprinted to answer the doorbell when it rang. She welcomed him in breathlessly, and he swooped her into the bedroom. The mattress bounced as she landed on it, but there was a funny thunking sound. Her boyfriend undressed, and when he got on the bed, she saw an arm flop out from under the bed. It was the body! Surely she had left it in the basement! What was it doing under the bed? If only she could get him to another location. She distracted her boyfriend so he wouldn't see it, and pleased by her eagerness, he got on top of her. As the mattress moved, the body beneath it seemed to be moving, too, so that their movements caused arms and legs to flop out. She moaned to try and conceal the noise. What was she going to do?

She awoke and could hardly believe her good fortune that this had all been a dream.

This dream combines two fairly prevalent dream themes: that of having to conceal a corpse, and of not having the right place or the right circumstances for sex. As morbid as they seem, corpse dreams may arise whenever there is pressure to edit the self for the tastes of a special situation, group, or person. The unexpected body represents whatever has to be tossed aside to be "okay" in the given situation. You can't really remember having done this, but there it is, and then you've got to respond to the same pressure in the dream and *get rid of incriminating evidence.* This dreamer is sure she has put everything in the basement (buried unacceptable things and any feelings she may have about doing so). But in the way of dreams, corpses don't stay where you put them, and of course emotions tend to flop out unexpectedly when you have sex.

Essentially there is nowhere for her to have sex at this point, because of course, the corpse is part of her and it will be wherever she is.

This dreamer was aware of the need to edit herself, to be careful, and to keep smoothing things along with her partner. Although the dream might have held a cautionary note, she stayed in the relationship for quite a while before it lost its luster.

Since dreams make emotions and issues into physical bodies and settings, sometimes the territory we roam represents trying to find a "place" in ourselves to put things.

Now on Sale at Nordstrom

One woman who was involved with a rather prominent older man felt self-conscious when they went out and people noticed them. She thought she felt their gaze flicker over her and think she was too young for him, but then, good for him. Whether this was true or not, it was an ongoing part of her experience, and something that she didn't know what to do with.

She dreamed that they were roaming in a shopping mall, people-watching and holding hands. They started noodling around in a corner and soon were seriously looking for somewhere to have sex. They tried an area near the changing rooms, but there was too much traffic. They tried an alcove near some offices, but it was too cold and the tiles were too hard.

Finally he found the perfect place, and they stretched out in an area that was softly lit, with soft fabric on the floor and mannequins nearby that created a feeling of privacy. They peeled off some of their clothes with relief and settled in. She only then looked over his shoulder to see that a happy crowd was gathering a few feet away. They were in a display window! She felt herself blushing, but didn't want to overreact. She whispered in his ear that she felt a little uncomfortable. He looked at the crowd and then looked back at her, smiling. He told her not to worry, who could blame them for staring? Then he removed more of her clothes and draped himself over her.

This scene illustrated the dreamer's confusion about just where to go with her feelings of being on display or exposed in this relationship. While they did have great chemistry, it was something that made her feel peculiar and vulnerable, as the dream suggests. No matter what she tries to do, she looks up and feels all eyes are upon them. But the dream gave her a new tidbit of information that was helpful. Maybe her boyfriend seemed to like the very attention that made her uncomfortable. His liking the same exposure she loathed heightened her uneasiness. No wonder she felt a little strain around this issue and an inability to discuss it with him. This issue was not insurmountable for them, and it certainly wasn't a deal-breaker. The dream did serve to put her on notice that these concerns were swirling around under the surface and that she might need time to explore them and resolve them on her own or with her partner.

When Is It My Turn?

We all seem to have pretty full lives these days, performing multiple roles and trying to play as hard as we work. Sometimes the very denseness of our lives intrudes on our sex lives and takes a toll.

A woman who returned home from vacation with her sister was greeted with the "to do" list from her family and the lets-make-up-for-lost-time sex with her husband. This was nice, but it came at the end of such a long day of dashing around, making everything work, and suspending tiredness that she tried to remember when she used to enjoy herself more.

That night she dreamed that she and her husband were driving in a convertible up a winding mountain road. The steeper the road became, the more the engine seemed to struggle to take them upward. Finally she told him she wanted to stop, not try to drive all day but to spend some time together that they could enjoy. They pulled over and registered at a little motel. When then went into the room, it opened into a much larger area than she'd expected, and as they moved through the back door, they found themselves in what seemed to be a European vacation spot. There was music playing, a fountain in a courtyard, and all sorts of colorful and warm people wandering by. They sat together and then began wandering around arm in arm.

This is really a dream about *finding* a place to make love and rediscovering how to be together. Sometimes dreams have a turning point, when everything goes wrong, or when a situation is retrieved. In this dream the "long hard journey" becomes a vacation when the dreamer simply and bluntly states her needs. Once she does that, the world expands, a little motel room has a portal to Europe, and two tired people become lovers wandering through romantic streets. Often dream scenes change with little explanation, but when a positive change occurs because of something said or done, it can be like a gift to the dreamer, suggesting a tactic to take in waking life that may set things moving in the direction you would like.

Dream Key #13

Find Your Place, Hold Your Space

There is a term used in some psychological and spiritual circles these days, and it is "holding a space" for something. Holding space means having mental and emotional room for something to be present, to be experienced. Therapists hold space for their clients and their issues; teachers hold space for students. It implies expanding some kind of inner resource so that things aren't made to be smaller than they need to be, and so that there is safe mental territory for something to be explored.

One of the tricks to understanding our dreams is to practice holding space for their exploration, and for our fears that if we do unravel them we might have to do something we don't want to do. If you stay with an image or a scene, it will speak to you. You just have to stop shouting how dumb it is, how meaningless or mistaken.

If you have a dream of not finding the right place for sex, or if your waking life seems too cluttered for intimacy or spontaneity, consider what it might mean for you to hold space for intimacy and passion again. Perhaps because of our current juggling act in life, women often crave encapsulated settings in which to feel themselves again. Here are some suggestions for holding space for passion.

1. Get away with your partner, somewhere sensual.

2. Do something blissful for your body at a spa; let it feel worshipped.

3. Only be a superhuman dynamo on alternate days of the week; on the off days set the bar at being human.

4. If you have a partner, make a list of all the sexy qualities they have and then read them the list.

5. If you don't have a partner, make a list of your most enjoyable sexual escapades and drink a toast to yourself.

6. Listen to music in a language you don't understand, so that the music can go directly to your center.

7. When you go to bed at night, ask for dreams to stir up your passions and give you some fun. If you keep asking, they will come.

CHAPTER FOURTEEN

Social Work Sex

It is intriguing how many women report sexual dreams of partners who are hurt, crazy, broken, or just bizarre. Since dreams can pluck fantasy partners from any corner of the globe, or create ideal lovers with perfect bodies and unlimited imaginations, why do so many women dream of being in an almost custodial role with a partner who is in need of help and support?

There are a number of possibilities with these dreams; they allow us to feel generous and sexy at the same time. A number of women reported dreams in which they felt stunningly beautiful and dripping with sexuality. Being a sexual goddess seems to be one of the things that makes the dreams fun. This may be why some women have dreams and even fantasies in which they are seen as more desirable than their partners.

One woman has a fantasy in which she becomes very famous and acclaimed for her work. She would have all sorts of offers from luscious men, but she would decline and stay with her current partner. He then would become worshipful and very grateful that she chose to stay with him. She loved to imagine them having sex under these circumstances: He would labor to please her and tell her he couldn't believe how lucky he was. She would wipe the sweat from his brow encouragingly and spend the day having multiple orgasms.

This fantasy shows the woman coming into her power and being recognized, not only by her partner but also by the people in her field. It also shows her enjoying being sought after by multiple partners, but not really having much interest in sampling the smorgasbord. What she really wants is greater power in her existing relationship, greater acknowledgment and importance. This fantasy also shows the connection between feeling valued and feeling sexy. Admittedly this is a bit of a cartoonlike scenario, but the core of it hints that the threads of feeling sexy are sometimes wrapped around the threads of feeling powerful and admired. For this person there is a touch of the rescuer, the loyal lover who could have anyone, but instead chooses to stick with her partner. He had better appreciate the choice, though, and make it worth her while.

In most dreams or fantasies of this sort, there is something overtly wrong with or strange about the partner, while the dreamer is rendered more beautiful, powerful and loving in contrast. She also becomes a sort of sexy saint by virtue of her decision to be with him. For many, there is something extremely erotic about this blend of sympathy, sex, nurturing, and power.

Varieties of Strange Love

Here are three glimpses into dreams where women act as sexual and emotional benefactors to partners who might be seen as flawed or problematic.

Android Sex

In this dream the woman was sitting upright on her bed, having sex with a very lifelike android. Like the character Data on *Star Trek: The Next Generation*, this android wanted very much to be human. They were sitting with their legs wrapped around each other while holding a Tantric posture, not really moving, just letting the tension build. He had a stunning penis that could expand or vibrate on command—very fun and versatile. She felt close to him and also very sorry for him. She looked at the flesh-colored plastic on his shoulder and thought how lifelike it appeared. His construction was really very good and clearly, he was "fully functional" as he so often claimed. He was, quite literally, a sex machine, but he wanted to be more; he wanted to be human. He hoped that by servicing her regularly, somehow the proximity would have an effect on him, and he would turn into a real person. She found the sex fantastic, because she was always the recipient, but she knew that the android was never going to get his wish, so she felt sad for him as well.

This dreamer was having a similar type of relationship in waking life at the time she had this dream. Her partner was a sexual virtuoso who was a bit lacking in social and life skills. They had an unspoken contract that had never been mentioned, but it went like this: They both felt she was doing him a favor by being with him, and in return he knocked himself out to provide mind-blowing sex. They both thought this was a great arrangement for a brief time, but she felt sad for him. On some level, he was hoping to be rescued or brought into the world. While the role of humanizing influence added to the sexual piquancy for her, it was not ultimately a relationship that had enough foundation to last. Why was her dream lover an android? Perhaps that image reflected her wish to be free to enjoy him without having custody of a real human heart. The movie *The Stepford Wives* poked fun at the fantasy of having android lovers who only exist to fulfill our superficial desires. The android lover used to be considered a male fantasy, but I suspect it is the fantasy of the busy person, who may at times feel there isn't enough time to always deal with relationship issues, schedules, and timing. Wouldn't it be handy to have a love machine in the closet that could do anything and would ask for nothing? It's a selfish fantasy, yes, but ultimately a fantasy about having fun without demands on time, responsibility, or emotion.

The Buried Torso

One striking dream involved the discovery of a man who had somehow been trapped in a concrete wall at a construction site. He was apparently surviving adequately, but only his lower torso was visible and accessible. The dreamer discovered him, lying on his back with his upper body hidden behind a concrete wall, his naked lower body stretched out. She tried to talk with him, but the wall muffled their communication. Somehow, in the magic manner of dreams, she knew that he was not suffocating. His upper body was on the other side, but she could not see or get to it. She tried to pull him free, but he was completely stuck. While they thrashed around, he developed an erection that was strikingly healthy-looking. A wave of heat washed over her, and she wanted to straddle him. A distant part of her mind seemed to watch this scene and to find it silly, but she couldn't help herself. She began fondling the trapped man, and it was clear from his response that he was pleased with the direction things were taking. She bent over and took some of his erection into her mouth briefly, just to let him know what was coming, and then lifted up her dress and straddled him. She was pretty sure she was not raping this poor fellow; she had a fleeting thought that if she couldn't rescue him, she could at least make them both feel good for a while. Then there was no more thinking, and she leaned her arms against the concrete wall as she let the heat have its way.

Though this was an enjoyable erotic dream while it was happening, the dreamer found this imagery kind of disturbing in retrospect. Why would she feel turned on by someone who was stuck in a wall? This was not related to any conscious fantasies; the dream came unbidden with specific detail. At the time of the dream, she was between relationships, so there may have been some sexual frustration building up. On examining the dream, she realized that a number of her relationships had been undertaken in pursuit of sex, and that often she didn't really want the relationships, as such, once she was in them. She was in the quandary many women face, of feeling that once she embarked on a sexual liaison with someone, it had to then be turned into a relationship. In many cases, she found herself responding to a visceral bond that flared instantly in the face of strong sexual chemistry. When she started having regular sex with someone, she also formed an attachment to them, which could be very powerful despite not having many of the "makings" of a workable relationship.

Dreams have a neat way of reflecting both our problems and our desires at the same time. The man in the wall reflected the problem she often faced in her personal life. She would hook up with someone "impossible" because of good chemistry, then when she wanted to communicate with him or he with her, it was as if there was a wall between them; they had no way of understanding or communicating with each other, except through sex. The wall also reflected a kind of waist-down accessibility that she found exciting. Here at last was someone she could enjoy without feeling the need to try and turn the contact into a relationship.

This dream is a good example of the way kooky, implausible scenes can shed light on real-life issues, hungers, and confusion. This dream also shows how we can have a number of differing "goals" in the psyche that are working toward fulfillment through our actions, decisions, fantasies, and dreams. When we hit a roadblock in waking life, the mind will focus on that and we will dream about it with various possible solutions or expressions. These dreams are part emotional expression, and part brainstorming for solutions.

This dreamer felt clearer after examining the man-in-the-wall dream, because it seemed to illustrate a dynamic that she was only aware of in the vaguest sense. She wanted "eventually" to find a life partner, but in the meantime she only wanted to have some fun with a series of "fuck buddies," so that she didn't go stir crazy while waiting for Mr. Right. But another part of her psyche seemed to be set on "auto-mate" so that any sexual partner would unconsciously be assessed and put on the conveyor belt leading to "improvements" and "making things work." Even though she didn't pick these partners as possible mates, some part of her seemed to rise up and start trying to set things in motion in that direction. This of course was a recipe for frustration, conflict, pain, and disappointment. When we make decisions with the part of our mind with which we are most familiar, the rational voice that we usually hear, we forget that other drives and agendas are alive and well inside us. We identify with a certain facet of ourselves, but it can be useful to remember that each of us is multifaceted, and we should factor in these elements even though they don't often stand at the microphone onstage when we are thinking things through.

While no clear-cut answer presented itself either through the dream or the exploration of it, she found it very useful to register just how strong were these two drives in her psyche. Proceeding with more awareness and consciousness is often all it takes to stop repeating a pattern that devours time and energy.

The Creature Feature

Do you remember the very old monster movies that focused on a sort of swamp creature that rose up out of a body of water? The title *Creature from the Black Lagoon* comes to mind. We seldom, if ever, hear any reference to such monsters (they have apparently gone out of style), but they do appear in dreams.

In one "creature dream" a woman was brought in to rescue a being that had been found living underwater in a swamp.

Officials were hosing off the creature, who was caked with stinking mud when she arrived on the scene. The creature was scaly like a reptile, but humanoid and obviously male. He was dazed and unable to communicate, and the officials didn't know whether to restrain him or take him to a hospital. The woman, who was kind of a victim-advocate social worker in the dream, took the creature home with her temporarily to see if she could establish any communication and rehabilitation.

Despite numerous baths, the creature always had a stench about him, but she hoped this would dissipate in time. He did have a sort of speech, mainly a loud barking voice with which he uttered strange critical comments. She felt that his criticism was a kind of code for some more normal communication, and she began taking notes on his utterances. Eventually the two became lovers (she could only imagine how lonely he must be, having lived in the swamp all that time). Once she adjusted to the feeling of his scales against her skin, and learned to breath through her mouth when he was close so that his odor was not so overpowering, they had an exciting sex life. He had a great deal of stamina and, presumably making up for lost time, seemed unable to get enough of her. Their genitals fit together with a series of clicks, like snap-on tools fitting together. Once in position, he was locked into her.

Everywhere she went, people warned her against keeping the creature with her for too long, or getting too attached to it. But secretly she had already decided to keep him and to continue working to reduce his smell and to teach him to speak more normally.

Upon reflection, this dreamer had little trouble recognizing her current partner in the creature, although his quirks were wildly exaggerated in the dream. He was not very sociable; he was highly critical and seemed fixated on her to an extent that she found very exciting. In turn, she was "hooked" by a sort of reforming instinct that had taken hold in her, and although her friends had tried to delicately point out his peculiarities and potential problems, she had decided to keep him and fix him up.

The dream pointed out that she even rationalized his grouchiness and criticism as "code for a deeper communication." What was the stench that seemed attached to the creature? She could only assume it was his negative, depressive atmosphere; something that drove other people away, but which she found acceptable as part of the whole lonely-creature scenario.

Many dreams are frankly offensive, if we wanted to evaluate them according to a standard of sensitivity or correctness. This dream makes the man look like a pathetic monster and the dreamer look like a compulsive rescuer. But the language of dreams is often exaggerated; the caricatures may not be attractive, and they are probably not *literally* truthful, either. Yet, like art, the highlighting or exaggeration makes a point we might not otherwise consider. This dream showed the dynamic at work under the surface of things, and showed how "social work" reflexes can not only take hold, but also heighten sexual intensity in some cases. If you have a dream like this, or you know someone who does, there may be a lot of apologizing, arguing, and defending going on. Accept the fact that dreams almost always exaggerate and amplify, particularly when exploring material that isn't part of our everyday awareness. It's possible to see the grain of truth in an exaggerated cartoon of a dream without feeling you have to respond to it with immediate action or a complete reversal of perspective. When our dreams and fantasies shed light on the patterns in our lives, then we have a chance to evaluate how and if we want to continue those patterns as we endeavor to create our futures. It is this lucidity that is one of the greatest gifts of reflecting on our erotic dreams.

The Frog Burial Ground

A woman once dreamed of having a backyard full of lawn ornaments, all of which were concrete frogs. It didn't take long for our dream group to wonder whether these frogs were little trophies of all the trial-and-error romantic adventures she'd had. She was a very social, sexy person who loved men and they loved her. But each time she embarked on a new relationship, her friends would think, "Where does she come up with these guys?" while she would describe him as being "full of possibilities." Perhaps because she had so much charm, warmth, energy, and make-things-work skills, she could easily turn on, engage, and manage a potential partner. Eventually she would feel cramped and annoyed, pick a fight with him, and break things off. This is how she got so many frogs in her backyard. This woman was not stupid or neurotic, not shallow or promiscuous or desperate. She was enthusiastic, really alive, and unaware of the pattern for a time. She would psychologically jump into a rowboat with a fellow, row them out to sea, and eventually notice she was exhausted and that she was doing all the rowing. She would then turn around and go back to shore and unload the fellow, surprised that he had never really pitched in.

Many women have taken a turn with this pattern, and it doesn't make us shallow or neurotic, nor does it mean that all men are frogs. It can be useful, though, to honestly examine how and when you engage in this pattern.

Dream Key #14

Where Do You Fall on the Continuum of Loving the Unlovable?

With a few exceptions, most patterns and symbols have both positive and negative potentials. It is up to the dreamer to honestly evaluate whether the tone of the dream and the patterns in waking life are manifesting in positive life-affirming ways, or are operating in negative, destructive ways.

Being helpful, being willing to see the beauty in someone who is not superficially "perfect" is a good thing; this is part of having a loving heart. Even being a born nurturer is a good thing. If we are fortunate, we all learn and grow in our relationships. Where this pattern can be negative is when it is unconscious and addictive, keeping people trapped in recurring behaviors that don't nourish them or allow them to grow.

In the last movie the late Audrey Hepburn made, she played an angel advising a recently deceased man to help his still-living lover to get over him and move on to love someone who could return her feelings and share her life on Earth. The angel said this was the right thing to do, and that to allow or encourage this woman to continue loving where it could not be returned would be *a waste of spirit*. I've always remembered that phrase, because it so perfectly fits behaviors and choices that not only lead us nowhere, but in a sense dishonor our uniqueness.

Answer the questions below and see if where you fall on the positive-negative continuum of social-work sex.

T F   1. I enjoy disappearing into the needs of my partner; it makes me feel safe and powerful.

T F   2. If I am in a relationship, I can't really do what I want until the other person is not around.

T F   3. I sometimes feel I am more "together" or evolved than the other person, and so expect less of them and more of myself.

T F   4. When I want to end a relationship, I can't seem to do it directly, so I wait and hope the other person will do it for me.

T F   5. I often find myself bound by the calendar, or by events. I can't have that talk because of the holidays, the family visiting, or his disappointment at work.

T F   6. My friends often seem to know what is going on with my relationships long before I do.

T F   7. When I take up with a new partner, I often have a series of dreams about old disastrous relationships the first week or so.

T F   8. Privately, I enjoy the fact that friends think I am nicer or more likable than my partner.

T   F   9. I like it when I'm with someone who treats others a bit harshly, but who is good to me because of our special connection.

T   F   10. Although I often complain to friends about my partner, and they give me all kinds of suggestions, I prefer to keep things steady rather than to act on any of those suggestions.

Add up the number of "True" answers.

Score 8–10. Strong pattern.

If you answered yes to most of these questions, it's possible that the social-work impulse is operating strongly in your psyche and in your relationships. This does not mean that you are messed up or that this is necessarily dysfunctional. But it does mean you would do well to *watch it* and consciously evaluate how this pattern is manifesting in your life and whether it is impacting your choices for good or ill.

Score 5–7. Moderate pattern.

You're probably a middle-of-the-road person when it comes to social-work-sex impulses. You're capable of an occasional rescue mission, but you also enjoy partnerships that don't involve rehab. It's possible you could still get stuck with something that doesn't serve you, or could take on a "project" without meaning to. Being honest with yourself and watching your dreams and fantasies will help you keep this pattern balanced and operating in a wholesome way in your life.

Score 1–4. Light pattern.

For you the social-work pattern is not all that sexy. You probably won't find yourself wondering how to extricate yourself from a connection, or starting over endless times with the same person who just disappointed you. You do have the ability to see potential in someone who may be rough around the edges, but you aren't going to sign up for years of compromise that doesn't work for you.

Whether you have a high, moderate, or low social-work-sex quotient, what matters is that you are fairly aware of your own profile, and that you are unafraid of evaluating how it is working for or against you. It is not useful to think of changing your nature, but instead to think of *knowing* your nature, and being aware enough to stay in the positive spectrum, where your gifts make your life better and enrich those you care about, rather than pull you into a black hole where you waste your spirit.

CHAPTER FIFTEEN

Interruptions

Interrupted sex is one of the classic contemporary sex dreams of women. (Men have it as well, but women are the grand champions of the interrupted-pleasure theme.) For women, interrupted pleasure comes in all varieties: Not only do we dream of people walking in and spoiling the moment sexually, we also dream of wishing we could just take a hot bath, or have more time in the shower without interruptions. While there are potentially a number of psychological themes involved in spoiled erotic moments, I also believe that these spoiled-sex themes are associated with the larger body of dreams in which women do not have time for their personal needs. As usual, the dreams are exaggerated, dramatized, and sometimes silly, but the underlying message of being derailed by lack of time or the needs of others is consistent.

Mom, Dad: This Isn't a Good Time . . .

A woman engaged to a businessman who frequently traveled cherished their time alone together. She also worried that his business commitments might be a strain on their relationship at some point, but she resolutely pushed that worry aside as she dealt with the more immediate pressures of planning their wedding.

During this "gearing up for marriage" period, she frequently had dreams that she and her fiancé were finally enjoying some luxurious time in the sack together. They had a great sex life and a great connection; it felt like something of a miracle to her to have everything she wanted in one person. In the dreams, just as they were getting rolling and the passion flared between them, one or both of her parents would appear in the doorway to ask her a question or make a comment. She and her fiancé would freeze, but the interrupting parent would simply lean in the doorway and speak as if nothing was happening. She would have been furious, but she was always so appalled that she would simply answer their question or reply politely and then hope they would go away. Usually at that point she would be so shaken that she would awaken from the aborted sex dream. In real life her parents would not be so crass, and she and her fiancé lived together alone. Like most interrupted sexual dreams, these were annoying as well as troubling.

There were three stressors affecting this dreamer that could have contributed to this theme. First, when we are on the threshold of a big change like getting married, our dreams tend to explore everything that could go wrong. Although she hadn't gotten to the dreams of the wedding itself going horribly wrong, her mind was exploring and exaggerating the tensions that were already undercurrents in her life. She wanted very much to build her own independent life, but somehow as she moved toward marriage, she felt herself and her fiancé saying and doing things that were like her parents. At the very time when she wanted to create something new, she felt herself enacting scenes from her history. Although what was said and done was not all that bad, it was troubling and bewildering to watch herself doing things that seemed to come out of her parents' playbook.

Second, her psyche was expressing what is called *dream vigilance*: guarding against anything that might sabotage or harm her primary relationship. We do not seem to have dreams of interrupted sex when we are having a fling; it is when we have discovered a profound connection, typically, that the mind begins to be truly vigilant and sensitive to influences that might intrude on our happiness. Whatever is most precious and sacred to you is always the one thing you wouldn't want to lose or have come to harm. For this dreamer, her relationship was that golden thing, and as she dealt with increasing tensions, her anxiety was expressed in dreams that showed that special relationship being spoiled and interrupted by those tensions.

Third, this dreamer had a legitimate worry regarding her relationship that she understandably was trying to squelch. Although she had fallen in love with this man knowing that his work required him to travel, it was in the back of her mind that this might not wear well over the long haul. But she wanted him, wanted to marry him, and didn't feel this was the right time to make demands or mess with his career. She didn't know if there would ever be a right time, and she also didn't want to be someone who said "I do," and who meant, "Yes—until I can get my way."

There was really nowhere for her to go with thoughts or feelings about the traveling issue. She felt she couldn't afford to get caught up in thoughts about it, so she didn't give herself the luxury of being clear about it within her own mind. Thoughts, feelings, and issues that have nowhere to go in waking life typically do arise in strange ways in our dreams. The less permission you have to *own* a thought psychologically, the more likely it is to come out in dreams. That doesn't mean that all your dreams are suppressed material, but it does mean that "unpopular" feelings and thoughts will pay you a surprise visit by night if you do not give them an appointment by day. I encourage people to sort through things with private candor, even if you decide not to share them with anyone. Just looking something squarely in the eye, going as far as you can with it, and then mentally shelving it to await further information and strategies can go a long way toward carrying it comfortably rather than carrying it with a cloud of tension around it.

You're Welcome to Join Us

Although most interruption dreams are about spoiled moments and feeling responsible for the feelings of others, fantasies of interruptions are considerably more fun. A woman who finally had a nice safe relationship after a series of tumultuous romances used to fantasize that one of her old outlaw boyfriends would stop by to have sex with her.

He would magically appear in the doorway of her bedroom, say her name softly, and then tell her to pull back the covers as he undid his belt and unzipped his pants. He quickly ran his hands and his mouth over her, then slid onto her as she wrapped her arms and legs around him. In a while her current, beloved-but-safe boyfriend would wander into the room. Instead of being angry, he would be curious and relaxed and lie down on the bed next to them. The outlaw fellow was equally unconcerned, and he slipped off her to make room for her boyfriend. As they moved together, it was hotter and more fun than usual. After they finished, they would look over and the outlaw boyfriend would be gone.

This fantasy gave the woman the best of both worlds, but it also helped her transition from the kind of partner she had been accustomed to, to the man she genuinely loved and preferred. Under the story line of coaxing and encouraging the safe new lover to be more adventurous and playful, she was really transferring her learned responses from one set of stimuli to another. She could simply have fantasized about rough sex with an edgy guy and left her lover out of it. Instead, at the end of the fantasy, the phantom from the past is banished, and she is having great sex with the one she really wants.

It's Not What You Think

One woman dreamed of having a tumble with the carpenter who was working on a remodeling project in her kitchen. She didn't have a thing for him particularly, though she had *noticed* that he was tan, sinewy, unfailingly polite, and smelled of soap and wood shavings in a way that was particularly nice.

In the dream they found themselves upstairs in the bedroom, and without much preamble they were soon wrestling playfully on the bed, then tearing off each other's clothes and kissing not so playfully. They were running their hands eagerly over each other and sliding closer together when a door slammed downstairs. There shouldn't be anyone home, and it could only be her husband. Damn. They leaped apart and hopped around frantically pulling on their clothes and straightening the bed. Too quickly they heard footsteps on the stairs and her husband's voice calling out. He came through the doorway and saw them standing on opposite sides of the room, trying to look casual, although they were out of breath and her shirt was on inside out.

Inspired by desperation, the dreamer then blurted out the cliché, "It's not what you think!" and attempted to convince her husband that she had brought the carpenter upstairs to have him give her an estimate on expanding the bedroom. Unfortunately, he didn't accept this explanation and turned on her quickly with bitterness. He kept saying, "I can't believe you would do this to me, I can't believe you would throw our life away." He stormed downstairs, and, although she tried to follow him and calm him down, she heard him start his car and drive away.

This woman found the dream very memorable because of the lovely sex scene with the carpenter, but also because of the nasty, guilty feeling she had at the end and when she awakened. She had a feeling of relief that it was only a dream and that she hadn't thrown her marriage away on a fling, and also a hazy sense that somehow the dream was important.

One way to cut to the core of a dream is to paraphrase the action it contains without describing too many details. When you read a brief movie review or the description of an episode in TV guide, they describe the whole story in a sentence or two. If you look at this dream in the broadest sense, it could be described in this way: A woman finds time to do something delicious and passionate and is interrupted by her mate, who accuses her of sabotaging their life together. This wasn't really a dream of wanting to cheat on her husband by messing around with a hunk in a tool belt, although the fact that he is a carpenter is significant. In dreams, carpentry, construction, and building all have to do with creating.

This woman had a small home business that had mush-roomed until she was faced with the choice of expanding it and seeing how much it might grow, or turning away business and keeping her life as it was. She wanted to expand, but her husband wanted her to keep the business on the margins of their life together. The dream hints that he felt threatened, perhaps not so much by demands on her time as by the pas-sion she had for her business. The dream also hints that she is feeling increasing pulled between her hunger to build the business and her sense that doing so would be a betrayal of her husband. Like many dreams, this one expresses the tension she is feeling and outlines the dynamics of her dilemma, but it does not appear to offer her a solution, at least in this presen-tation. The only hint we have of a possible strategy is her at-tempt to communicate with the jealous husband. She tries to tell him, "This isn't what you think, I don't want to betray you or hurt you, I want to expand something."

It takes a lot of stability and confidence not to be thrown off balance when one partner wants to change significantly. It is possible this dreamer was feeling forced to go underground with her hunger because she didn't feel the climate was safe for an honest exploration of plans and possibilities. While a number of spouses go underground with their interests and passions because they don't go over well in their relationship, this tends to heighten the other spouse's feeling of being cuckolded in some inexplicable way. Most of the time, these tensions are swimming around beneath the conscious thoughts of both parties; none of this is planned and no one is particularly at fault. Dreams of interrupted passion in which the spouse is the spoiler are sometimes reflecting this conundrum of primary relationships.

In other cases, the interrupting party actually represents a side of the lover that tends to create uneasiness or reduce passion.

Okay, Dirtbag, Step Away from the Girl

It seems inevitable that people of differing backgrounds and styles will find each other irresistibly attractive. The very differences that create intoxicating sparks can create friction once people get down to the work of seeing how their lives can fit together. One self-described wild woman fell in love with a police officer, and they both felt they had found their soulmate. In the beginning they found their dramatic differences in style and thinking hilarious, and every newly discovered divergence was a source of wonderment and humor.

After a time, however, the wild woman began to feel a little less wild, a little less sexy, and a little less in love. She adored the policeman, she reminded herself, but he did seem to have an awful lot of *rules*.

One night she dreamed of being with her lover outside under the stars. They were making love on a blanket up in a high meadow as they had done in real life during the summer. It was cool and they were keeping each other warm with activity and heat. She was on top, pretending to hold him down and moving slowly in circles. He apparently got frustrated and rolled them over so he was on top and could speed things up. She laughed, and then stopped laughing as a wash of deepened sensation left her breathless. Just then a booming voice as if through a megaphone blasted both of them: "Step away from the girl!" They froze. The voice repeated: "Get off her, dirtbag! Step away from the girl!" A light shone on them, and they both realized that the police were there, and were assuming they had stumbled upon a rape in progress. She opened her mouth to explain that she wasn't being raped, but only a squeak of sound came out. As she struggled to speak in her dream, she made real-life sounds that awakened her from the dream.

It was not hard for this woman to reduce this dream to a single description. "Passion with my partner is interrupted by the arrival of *law enforcement* personnel." Notice that the instruction made through the bullhorn was to step away from the girl. Although we can only speculate, this hints that her psyche was picking up an undercurrent of feeling that her lover was going through a phase of feeling some need to distance himself from her, to step back. From her perspective, it is much easier to read that what interrupts or ruins some of the passion in the relationship is the sense of rules and authority. When they had met it was as if the policeman were saying, "Let's break all the rules together," a territory the dreamer knew well and was only too happy to share. But as they settled into a relationship over time, much of it was shaped by the policeman's understandable sense of order and respect for guidelines. To a woman whose erotic sensibility appreciated the exploration of taboos and the release of inhibitions, this was like trying to swim in quicksand.

Dreams depict feelings as physical actions. Connection is often depicted as intercourse while ambivalence or hurt is depicted by physical distance, or sexual disappointment. Dreams exaggerate our disappointments and confusion, turning them into memorable physical dramas that improve dream recall while allowing our complicated feelings to run their course. Your dreams not only reflect the quality of the connection you're making in waking life, they also track the phase (new, old, etc.) that the relationship is in and how that is adding to the mix. Sexual and romantic relationships tend to bloom in an initial phase of euphoria and intoxicating sex. In this euphoric phase nothing is wrong, and everything is delicious. When this phase gives way to "being in a relationship" there is usually a stretch of time when horrible disappointment ensues, passion is blighted by reality, and it appears that things will never work out. The sex is still reasonably good, so you decide to hang in there until it really dries up, but secretly you've moved the relationship from category A (this is it) to category B (this is it until the real thing comes along).

Fortunately this phase of disappointed realism also gives way, and when you move through it, like emerging from a tunnel, there are sometimes possibilities evident that were not imagined during the earlier stages. This dream, as you might guess, arose during the disappointment phase of a relationship. It showed passion blighted and love cringing in the spotlight of Gestapo-like authorities who ordered the two to separate. This also shows how dreams will use different characters to play the part of different sides of a single person's personality.

The partner on the blanket represents the things she connects with in her lover. The policeman with the bullhorn represents the "rules" and authoritarian qualities that she doesn't like and which she feels are dampening their connection.

You could analyze this dream and interpret it to say: This relationship isn't working; the two people are too different. Or you could interpret it to say: There are some inhibiting factors that are trying to move from unconsciousness to consciousness so they can be properly evaluated. This dream arose during the phase of shattering disappointment, so it was naturally reflecting the tone of that phase. The dreamer in question decided on a wait-and-see interpretation. It does seem like a probable twist of fate that an outlaw and a law-man would fall in love and have great potential lessons for each other as well as passion to share.

Dream Key #15

Guidelines for Evaluating Interrupted Passion

Figuring out what a dream is *about* is only half the work of interpretation. The other very important half is evaluating the implications of the dream; this is the hard part, but without it, dreamwork can be just a game. In the above example, the dream was pretty clearly reflecting the dreamer's frustrations with the relationship. But evaluating the dream for its possible value to her in making decisions, having patience and greater understanding was the important part.

Keep in mind that your instinct is the best tuning fork of

accuracy you have with respect to deciphering a dream and evaluating its implications. These guidelines are derived from probabilities and are only presented as a reference.

1. Interruption scenes can reflect inhibiting factors in your current relationship. The real-life intrusion may be a set of ideas, the traditions of your family of origin (or just their vibes wafting into your bedroom), the proximity and responsibilities of parenthood, or a change in one or both partners. Typically the intruding factor will be depicted as a *person* who barges in, causes trouble, or spoils the moment. If something is dampening the heat between you two, it may take a while to notice it in real life. Your dreaming mind is going to pick up on this and be bothered by it before you do. This side of your psyche thinks your sex life, and your primary relationship, are the gold in Fort Knox; anything that messes with this part of your life is going to be highlighted and presented in a dream production big time.

2. Some erotic interruptions represent influences in your life that are clamping down on your creative, professional, or spiritual passion. To the dreaming mind, passion is passion; juice is juice. If it turns you on, makes you feel alive, sets something in you on fire, its probably going to be reflected as a sex dream. For whatever reason, dreams make everything physical. If you're going to do a production about absolute passion and you've got to make it physical, how do you do it? Well, the best way is to do it with sex.

There is nothing too shocking or taboo to be used in a dream symbolically. One woman who started volunteering at a local church felt a spiritual passion rising in her. She had a dream that she was shakily disrobing a priest when some friends came upon them, and they flew apart as if they were committing the ultimate sin. She was feeling passionate about her newfound sense of community and a little embarrassed and apologetic that she had found a "home" in what she considered such a traditional place. She found herself downplaying her enthusiasm to her friends, treating the situation as if she had a secret lover. It wasn't cool. It was a bit of a departure, and she had nowhere to go with this sense of passion. It was dampened by her fears of what her friends might think.

3. Some interruption dreams literally suggest sexual techniques that might please you. If you do something in an erotic dream that turns you on (which is safe), and it gets aborted in the dream, you may want to try some version of it in waking life. Dreams often imply literal suggestions to improve life, such as getting more rest, exercising, and driving more carefully. Sexual dreams sometimes get very explicit about positions, oral sex, foreplay, different locations, and moods. Sometimes just a fresh perspective or a mini-vacation can change something routine into something much more exciting. In some of our dreams I suspect that our interruptions are the mind's way of saying: look at how much fun this would be, don't just put on your workaholic hat and then try to have dynamite sex while your mind is still racing at the office. Try this little bit of a change and see how it feels.

4. In some cases the interrupting person represents a side of your own personality, or a side of your partner's personality. I once had a dream that a small gnomelike man was racing around my bed in which my partner and I had fallen asleep.

The snarly little man was saying: Get up, get to work, keep busy, do something, don't just lie there! I sat up in my dream and said: "What are you doing? Who are you?" He laughed an evil little laugh and said, "I'm not talking to you; I'm talking to him. I keep him busy, that's my job, I keep him busy. Hahahahahaha." This daunting little dream showed my sense that my partner was not only very productive, but was perhaps haunted by something that kept him busy, sometimes to the point of being lifted out of his own life.

The simplest way to get a handle on your dream is to paraphrase it in a single sentence or two as if you were writing a movie review. Then consider whether the interruption is providing commentary on your current relationship, another kind of passion that's being suppressed, is offering a sexual prescription, or is sorting through the effects of different sides of your or your partner's personality.

CHAPTER SIXTEEN

Apparent Incest

Few things are as freaky as having a sexual dream about a family member. In addition to the creepy factor, such experiences raise dark questions as well. Are you recalling a hidden memory of abuse so horrible that you've blocked it out? While some people do have buried memories, most people seem to be pretty well aware of early abuse. If you are sure that the literal explanation for a dream makes no sense, then relax and stop worrying about that. Remember that dreams are not politically or socially correct: If a family member is the most apt figure to depict something, then a family member it will be.

Sex with Dad

One woman reports that she has married a man who is in some ways similar to her father. However, while her father was not the most emotionally available person, her husband is devoted and kind. Still, he has shades of the workaholic in his personality, as did her father. What troubles this woman is that she often has dreams of having sex with her dad, and that partway through these dreams she pulls away, disgusted and horrified. There was no sexual abuse in her family, of that she is sure; so why these intermittent themes of incest?

After some exploration, this woman concluded that her dreams of intimacy with dad are expressions of her frustrations in her current relationship. The dreams illustrate the tricky dance of being married to someone who pushes her buttons because he is like her parent, yet who in many ways heals early wounds of neglect, because he is attentive and emotionally healthy. She believes that sometimes she does not give her husband a chance, because she has a kind of automatic response to him that stems from early disappointments with her father. Sometimes she shuts down, when her husband would be glad to try and work things out together. When she searches her heart to see if such response is warranted by current events, she has to say no. There is nothing insurmountable or unhealthy in the marriage, it is more the case that she distances herself from her husband without consciously knowing she is doing it.

When we look at the dream symbolically, it shows her essentially trying to have a relationship with her parent, through her relationship with her husband. When the result is positive, it can be miraculously healing, but when the result is frustrating, it can keep them both locked in a script that has more to do with history than current events.

Considering the sexual dream triangle, the dream does seem to hold important clues to what she wants, what she doesn't want, and how she can make things work. It shows the dreamer wanting closeness, intimacy, and fulfillment. What she doesn't want is to constantly have her loving relationship with her husband contaminated with all the echoes of her early wounds from her father. How can she make this work? By pulling away from her father. The recurring dreams essentially show her saying: "Yuck! I don't want to be making out with Dad! How disgusting!" This is a symbolic way of saying: *Take a look at this pattern. This is not something that you would do if you were conscious of it, right?* The very unsettling series of dreams came with a gift of suggesting that she become more conscious of this pattern and therefore take steps to let go of it. Tangled and unconscious material is hard to deal with, particularly when you don't know it is there, and if you do glimpse it, it seems so ugly and bizarre that it's alarming to even try and figure out what it represents.

This dream, like many dreams containing incest themes, has a lot of shock value. It takes an act of will to examine the possible meaning of such a dream, but usually there is great value in dreams that send us a zinger like this. This dreamer developed a self-statement that she used to set her intention. She would simply think to herself: "This is not my father, this is my husband, and today is a new day. We are free to build our relationship on our own terms." As simple as it sounds, self-statements can be very powerful and help us to stay lucid and current in our thinking. The more time goes by, the more free she feels from the past, and it may be that these initially troubling dreams had something to do with moving her into the greater emotional freedom and fulfillment.

Masturbating Dad

One dream that stands out to me was that of a woman who came to me upset because she had a vivid dream of masturbating her father. We talked it over, and she was certain that there was no sexual activity or incest in her childhood. So, freed from literal translations, we considered symbolism. In contemporary terms when someone is yanking your chain, or jerking off, it sort of implies someone is leading you on, or making you feel good but not necessarily being honest. This dreamer was, in fact, having a relationship that she was hiding from her father. When she talked to her father long distance on the phone, she told him all sorts of things that she knew he wanted to hear, but she did not tell him about the relationship that was most important to her at that time, because she knew that it was something he would never appreciate or approve of. This made her feel guilty and strange, because she was close to her dad, and really wanted to confide in him and share the fact that she was in love. But instead, she just "stroked him" and felt as if she was telling a lie by leaving out such a huge part of her life. It made her feel dirty—as if she was letting down her lover, her father, and herself just to keep things pleasant.

The dream seemed to be reflecting her sense of taking the low road on this issue and of feeling a bit soiled by the whole thing. However, she was relieved to find an explanation for the dream that did fit her circumstances and her emotional undercurrents. She decided for the time being to hold off on talking to her father while she waited to see if the relationship was going to last and be a part of her life for years to come.

Incestuous Friendship Encounters

Sometimes we have dreams that involve close friends, or the spouses of best friends who are so close to us in real life that we think of them as family. When we have a sizzling dream encounter with them, it not only worries us in terms of betrayal, but it also feels nasty because of the emotional incest. These dreams can be almost as troubling as family-incest dreams, because they are just as taboo but for different reasons.

One woman had repeated dreams about her best friend's husband and found these very disturbing. She thought he was cute and lovable, but he really wasn't someone she would pursue, even if they both were free and available. So why the erotic scenes? When she examined the dreams for what they told her about what she wants, she felt pretty clear that she knew what was going on. Her friend's husband was one of those "sensitive guys" who understands about buying cards and flowers at the right times, bringing his wife a hot water bottle when she has cramps, and generally being tuned in to her needs. The dreamer likes he-man types, finding the masculinity and apparent strength a turn-on. But partway through her relationships, she starts to feel lonely and misunderstood. She wanted to settle down and get married (another possible reason why she "borrowed" her best friend's husband in her dreams), but she seemed to be picking men she really didn't want and then rejecting them. The dreams helped her understand that by picking prospective husbands exclusively for their washboard abs, she was perhaps overlooking some more subtle qualities that she would find emotionally nourishing and more enduring.

When she examined the sexual dream triangle to see the implications of these dreams, she said: "I want to get married, and I want to be emotionally nurtured to some degree. I don't want to be lonely down the road, when it becomes clear the attraction of opposites is the only thing we had in common. What do these dreams imply about getting what I want? Begin considering the potential value of men who have different qualities than the action-hero types that I usually pick." As simple as this sounds, the dream implications had never occurred to her consciously before.

Engaged to My Brother

A woman was troubled by a series of dreams in which she was engaged to marry her brother. The dreams were not vivid in terms of erotic content, but she was troubled by the implications. She had a close, normal relationship with her brother, and was unclear why the dreams were so persistent.

Often dreams only begin to make sense when we step back from them and describe the theme from a distance. She described her brother as a wonderful fellow, who was protective and condescending, as if he continued to view her as a child who needed his advice even though they were each successful adults. When she asked herself whether there was any person or any energy in her life currently that was protective and somewhat condescending, she realized that her significant other was in fact very much in that mold. He was several years older than she, and more successful as well. Although she always dismissed it, she often felt he was being a bit patronizing to her and that he underestimated both her intelligence and her nerve. She found herself hoping that as she succeeded and gained recognition, he would somehow acknowledge her accomplishments and "see her" as more of a whole person. What emerged, over time however, was that they had something of an unconscious contract in their relationship. It felt as if the basis of their closeness was that he would always be in a bit of a one-up position, giving her advice and patting her on the shoulder. While the majority of their connections are close and very positive, she was appreciative that her dreams had pointed out the parallel with her protective brother who seems to see her as less than fully adult. She is going to give the relationship time and see how things play out.

Fantasy: The Sexy Brother-in-Law

How many women have wondered to themselves if perhaps they picked the wrong brother in the family to fall in love with? A number of women say that their charming brother-in-law is often a favorite fantasy figure for them. Taboo enough to feel naughty and hot, yet someone they have real emotional feelings of affection for as well.

In this fantasy there is some bizarre thing that throws you together with your brother-in-law. Like an adolescent confessing his crush, he suddenly discloses to you that he's longed for you for years, and you fall into each other's arms, discarding clothes and consummating your forbidden passion.

There is nothing quite as promising as someone who gives you positive recognition, but rarely any criticism or real-life friction. Typically, a well-liked brother-in-law is just such a person. He likes your cooking, he may seem to admire your appearance and envy his brother, and there is a rosy glow to your encounters with him. In fact, he is very much like your husband or significant other, before he started to take you for granted.

I believe the brother-in-law fantasy is the most natural thing in the world; it manifests in dating years as fantasies about your boyfriend's best friend. While best friends aren't biological brothers, they are often *emotional* brothers, and dreams tend to depict *qualities* in people and in life roles. When the marriage or partnership is mostly positive, the brother-in-law fantasy is in one sense a reinforcement of all the things you find attractive in your mate, while supplying the admiration, newness, and forbidden sparks that may feel like they are on the wane.

If you sometimes fantasize about a brother-in-law type, pay attention to what seems to make the fantasy satisfying. Does he seem to admire and understand you, anticipating your needs and preferences? Or is there just a tug of chemistry that you probably will never explore in real life that is delicious to think about in fantasy? At some point routine activities with your mate or partner can feel like work, while get-togethers with the brother-in-law are usually special occasions at least to some degree. Thus, in one sense, the brother-in-law theme gets merged with the somewhat happy prospect of weekend gatherings, dinners out, and fun time off. This fantasy may have very personal triggers, but one general thing that coincides with this fantasy is a hunger for time off, time away from routine, and time dedicated to pleasure and fun.

Dream Key #16

Discovering the Message in Incest Themes

1. Give yourself permission to work with this theme as you would any other dream, without judging or being put off by the subject matter. Remember dreams are a "free zone" without politics, propriety, or rules. Remember, too, that most dreams are *symbolic* and are not *symptoms*.

2. There are two predominant ways incest symbolism works: The first is that the sexual partner represents someone close to you in waking life, like a lover who has the same sort of sense of humor as your dad or your brother. You may feel automatically at ease and free with your lover partly because you "get" his humor, you're already tuned in and have jumped into a level of intimacy that is ahead of the ordinary dating time line. It feels like you already know this person, like you have come home. It probably won't register consciously that you are feeling especially comfortable because you're dating someone so much like your relative. But your dreaming mind will get it right away, and your dreams will reflect it. Just remember, you aren't attracted to this person because you have a thing for your relative, you feel comfortable and safe because

you feel familiar, and because this personality profile is something you already know how to love. The second way incest dreams work is to reflect a sort of emotional compromise that is confusing and disturbing, like the woman who lied to her dad and then dreamed of masturbating him. Incest dreams also appear when family systems have rather enmeshed and overly close traditions of behavior—not so much in physical terms but in terms of sharing information, sharing money, or operating according to childhood rules long into adulthood. Even when these families are fairly positive and wholesome, members still can feel strange and not know why, or feel trapped because any question of the rules is impossible; there is no right of refusal.

3. One useful way to work with incest themes is to reduce them to very simple forms and fill in the blanks. Instead of saying your dad or your brother, say *dad-like energy*, or *brother-like energy*. This may be enough to put the meaning of the dream into a context for you. For example:

In my dream I am intimate with . . .
During the dream this seems . . .
My overall reaction in the dream is . . .
When I awaken, I feel . . .

Is this a theme of some kind of boundary violation? Is it about someone in your real life with qualities similar to a family member? Is it about some sort of line that is being crossed in a part of your life that makes you uncomfortable?

4. If you have a handle on what the dream is reflecting, does this incident, as disturbing as it may be, provide some clue or insight into what posture you want to take with the situation in waking life? Are you going to proceed watchfully, ask for some candid conversation, or simply make tactful choices that will move you into a place where you feel more autonomous?

CHAPTER SEVENTEEN

Undesirable Partners

With all the interesting and sexy people who *could* show up in your dreams, why would you dream about someone you don't like and aren't attracted to? This seems like a waste of a perfectly good sex dream; it doesn't make sense that your mind would drop in someone so unappealing. The action may be fairly pleasing during the dream, but the next day you may be worried that your taste has suddenly taken a very weird turn.

One woman who had been promoted from administrator to marketing representative dreamed that she was spending the night with one of the other salespeople whom she particularly disliked. She described him as a rude, cutthroat sales "star," who treated people like dirt unless they were customers. But in her dream this fellow was a sexual dynamo who pushed all her buttons and made her feel uninhibited and alive. When she awoke, she wondered if maybe she'd been wrong about him, maybe there was some potential there, some attraction. But when she went to work, he was just as repulsive as ever. He was rude, arrogant, and just not her type. The dream did not seem to reveal any hidden attraction for her coworker, but it did coincide with her own change of roles in the organization. She was now "in bed" with the sales force; she was one of them. Not only was she doing work that was new and different, but her job also made her tingle when her powers of persuasion enabled her to succeed. Her ability to make money was now theoretically unlimited, and this brought a surge of power and possibility that was quite a rush. Sometimes she felt herself "getting off" on her ability to make things happen and to get people to buy what she was selling. Her dream night in the sheets with the rude salesman seemed to parallel her thrill with her own powers. Success is intoxicating sometimes; it's fun and seductive. But why did her mind select the salesman she liked the least, instead of one of the many who seemed friendly and well rounded? Perhaps it was because her psyche was warning her to stay awake and not to lose her way. The fellow in question was almost like a cartoon character, stepping on people he felt were unimportant while kissing up to potential clients. Most people thought he was rude and pretty nasty, while his customers thought he was great because he went out of his way to charm and flatter them.

After she got over the shock of the dream, and understood that it was about her career and not some secret yearning for the slimy guy, she found the dream valuable. It seemed to be celebrating her talent to succeed while it also cautioned her to stay aware of the difference between persuasion and exploitation, charm and phoniness. It is unlikely that she would ever turn into an exploitative stinker, but perhaps the dream was just balancing the scales of her enthusiasm by cautioning her not to become so singular in her focus that it seemed nothing else mattered as much as success.

Fantasy: Great Sex with a Revolting Guy?

Not many of us fantasize about people we don't like or find unattractive, but there can be something freeing about a fantasy partner that you wouldn't really want for keeps. One woman told me of reading a historical novel in her teens that has stayed with her because it formed the basis of an enduring fantasy.

In the novel's convoluted plot, the heroine was forced to marry a wealthy older man, though she was in love with a rugged highwayman. In a strange twist, the unwanted husband was rather a stud. Though she really couldn't stand him and plotted to run away someday, in the meantime he drove her crazy in bed, try though she might to avoid responding to him. Setting aside the absurdity of the plot for a moment, consider how the bizarre situation led to the sexual freedom of the heroine in the story. She cannot say no to the husband, and though she longs for her true love, she's killing time having multiple organisms with the wealthy beast she's married to. For the already sex-obsessed teenager reading the story, this was an interesting premise: being trapped by a wealthy sexual virtuoso didn't seem like a bad fate, really. This has proven a useful fantasy in later life, principally because it links the occasion of (initially) unwanted sex with the surprising capacity for pleasure. This woman said that when she's tired, cranky, or not in the mood, she can sometimes transform boring sex by remembering that story, and pretending she is the hapless heroine servicing the insatiable husband. This is more stimulating than just being a tired, modern-day woman burdened with worries at the end a tough day, and it seems to carry her across a bridge from reluctance to relaxation and pleasure.

The Bare Essentials

One college student had a quirky dream about one of her professors. He was an attorney who was also an instructor. Although she admired him, he wasn't exactly her style, and she didn't particularly think she'd like an older man as a partner.

But in the dream, as they were talking, she felt a sudden rush of attraction toward him. She felt herself getting hot and her face was becoming flushed. She caught him looking at her chest with such fixity that she glanced down at herself, and saw that one of her breasts was exposed, just hanging out of her blouse. Hmmm. How long had she been going around like that? Her teacher raised his eyes to meet hers, and cleared his throat. "Are you trying to flirt with me?" he asked mildly. She was suddenly embarrassed and said, "No, not at all, that's just a wardrobe malfunction." She awoke from the dream thinking it was quirky and cute, obviously a take-off on the incident with Janet Jackson's costume that had made the news that year.

Upon reflection, she could come up with no reason why she would dream of feeling hot over her instructor, or why she would be unaware of flashing a breast at him. Was something about her sticking out plainly for everyone to see, while she was completely unaware of it? Then she realized that one aspect of the dream was true: She was flirting with the idea of applying to law school, and her love of the professor's class was one reason why she thought she would like to pursue the profession. But every time she came close to filling out the paperwork, she became self-conscious and self-doubting, and put the forms away in a drawer. As she got close to pursuing the thing that turned her on, she would think: "Who do I think I am? Just because I like it, doesn't necessarily mean I can do it." The pattern in the dream was very much like her inner dialogue; the recognition of passion, flirting with the idea of exploring it, followed by a feeling of embarrassment and avoidance.

Sometimes our hunger for meaningful work, a cause, or activity is depicted in a dream as erotic desire. When a dream is working with material that is visceral or heartfelt, the dream is likely to be "juicy," too, and many times sex is the theme. In such cases, nudity or partial nudity can represent vulnerability or truth, or even a kind of bare "essential" self. The bare-breasted dream held a kernel of truth that left the dreamer thinking about possibilities. It is useful to ask yourself if a dream or fantasy hints at something you didn't know before. In this case, the dreamer realized two things: Her longing for law school was stronger than she'd realized, and she would have to be on the lookout for a sense of near shame about her ambition, interests, and goals. At that point it felt more natural to back away from her passions than to move forward and explore their promise. Knowing this was her tendency, she felt emboldened to push herself to send in her applications and see what happened.

Even Stranger Bedfellows

One of the reasons dreams are valuable to explore is because they have a core of truth running through them. Often this truth is shrouded with symbols, bizarre juxtapositions, or shocking themes. Unless a dream makes sense literally, don't worry that you have some secret thing for zombies or aliens; assume those partnerships have symbolic meaning and look at the overall plot of the dream to see what it reveals.

One woman said that she had an elaborate dream about being from an alien planet. In the dream she had been sent to Earth on a mission to learn about human beings, and to take what she learned back to the home planet so that they might be more compassionate and understanding. The dream seemed to cover her lifetime thus far, with the interesting twist that she was taken up on an orbiting ship regularly to visit her alien friends and have sex with them. The sex was pretty great, although a little weird, since they were sort of like insect-people. At the end of the insect-alien conjugal orgy, the space people informed her that they wouldn't be picking her up for any more visits with them, because they wanted her just to live her life as if she were a human being. She was not to worry about the fact that she would never feel quite like other people; her job was not to try to be like everyone else, but to watch, learn, and absorb what she could about love and compassion.

As bizarre as this dream sounds, it was a pivotal moment for the dreamer. A profound introvert, she had long felt "alienated" from the mainstream of life and had struggled long and hard to be more like other people. The dream suggested that she was never meant to be like everyone else, she was meant to be different, and that in her nonconformity lay her strength. She was here to learn, rather than to endeavor to become like everyone else. Although the dream was initially memorable for its great sex with insect people, it turned out to be profound in its essential truth. It suggested that if she freed herself from the obsession with how different she felt, her life would be more interesting and fulfilling. This may sound like a one-of-a-kind dream, but themes of being from "somewhere else" are more common than you might expect. Whenever I tell this story, I get responses from people who have had very similar dreams.

The Payoff to Understanding Erotic Dreams

If you're not used to thinking about dreams, they pretty much seem like someone put your day in a blender and turned it on high. What emerges at night seems randomly arranged with only occasional flickers of plot. But if you pay attention to dreams for a while, they are amazingly consistent, possessing a kind of syntax of their own. While there are *always* individual qualities and reasons for particular dreams, there are, in a sense, rules of genre, just as there are in literature and film. Nightmares operate in a certain typical fashion, as do anxiety dreams. Women's erotic dreams tend to reflect the angles of a triangle within the psyche: One corner is what you want, the other corner is what you don't want, and the third corner is how you can best *get* what you want. As I tell my clients, erotic dreams are not always about sex, but they are always about passion.

I Didn't Feel a Thing

Some partnerships in our dreams are puzzling because in waking life, we wouldn't select that person for a relationship or even a fling. But other dreams provide strange erotic episodes when idyllic opportunities prove disappointing.

One fairly common dream is that of gearing up for a charged sexual encounter with someone who seems attractive, sexy, and available. The timing is right, the foreplay is fun, and you're ready for more. But for some reason, when it comes time for coitus, you just don't feel anything. You can't very well say, "Um, are you there, are you *doing* anything?" The partner seems to be having a fairly interesting time, but it's as if there's nothing down there but a breeze. Allowing room for individual interpretations, why would so many women report this type of theme? On its most basic level, the theme seems to suggest that something expected, anticipated, and desired is missing. Whether the "something missing" has to do with sexual activity or something more abstract is perhaps an individual question. Some dreamers have reported they believe the dream is a reflection of a somewhat unfulfilling sex life, while others have said they believe the dream hints at a kind of disconnect from their own "masculine" potentials.

The Case of the Vanishing Penis

One prevalent version of the "nothing doing" dream is that of the partner with the vanishing genitals. Interestingly this dream is one that women seem to have in clusters: It recurs for a few years and then seems to go away. In this dream you're with a fairly yummy fellow (usually fictitious) and you're having a slippery, sweaty encounter leading to its inevitable and lovely conclusion. But just when you can't wait anymore and you reach down to move things along in your helpful way, you discover that his penis has suddenly disappeared. Shocked out of your poise, you sit up and look the situation over. Sure enough, like a cartoon that's been erased, it's just gone! For the majority of women, the dream essentially hangs up there; you get frustrated and wake up. In some cases there's a bit more struggle, as if you refuse to believe a perfectly nice anatomical part could just evaporate like that. One resourceful dreamer eventually discovered the organ somewhere in the sheets, it apparently having fallen off somehow.

What do our dreams of lack of sensation or evaporating genitals imply? A number of women who report these dreams say they had them when they were in a somewhat uninspired relationship, or when they had no relationship at all. So on one level, it's possible that these dreams reflect a sense of frustration, that there really wasn't a fulfilling connection there at the time. On another level I wonder whether these dreams reflect a lack of available masculine energy or support as well.

Dream Key #17

Measuring Erotic Sensations

If you've ever had an injury that took you to the emergency room or doctor's office, you may have been asked to rate your pain on a scale of 1 to 10 with 1 being the least and 10 being the most. As annoying as this question may be when you're hurting, there is great value in rating something as subjective as pain or feeling. It gives you a point from which to begin assessing the situation and thus know how best to respond to it.

If you can recall an erotic dream of yours now, use it to respond to the following questions and begin to get a handle on measuring your erotic sensations.

1. On a sexy scale of 1 to 10, how physical and palpable were the sensations in your dream? Generally dreams that have a high sensation ratio, such as 7 and up, are really about sex and what satisfies you. If you rate the sexy scale of your dream fairly low, it's likely the dream may be more symbolic in nature. It may be about something else in your life that you feel passionate or turned on about, or just something you are connecting with in a positive way.

2. Consider the dream in the most general of terms. If it doesn't make sense in literal terms, then consider the symbolic theme. Are you connecting with someone who has qualities you admire? Are those qualities something that you are trying to develop in your own life?

3. If you think of the dream in terms of the sexual dream triangle in your psyche, does it have any implications for you? Remember that some dreams comment on what you want, others dramatize what you don't want, while others provide clues on how to navigate through a transition or make a wise choice. If your dream were a movie being reviewed, would the morale of the story be "Follow your heart!" or "Proceed with caution!"?

Remember: Let go of how weird the dream might appear on first examination. Focus on what it may reveal in terms of what you want, what you should avoid, and how you can move forward in your life. If there are parts that you still have questions about, put them on the margins for now. Stepping away from pushing an interpretation usually lets the truth pop into your mind when you least expect it.

PART FOUR

The
Mystical Side

CHAPTER EIGHTEEN

PSI Sex

Dreams are often our first psychic experiences. They sometimes come true, or appear to, and they are often part of a confluence of events tied up together. For people who don't routinely remember dreams, a strange sexual encounter that smacks of the supernatural will almost certainly be remembered, sometimes for years. But who do you talk to about these experiences? What if someone who wasn't there came into your room and had sex with you?

It Was a Dream, Right?

One woman dreamed that she was in her bed sleeping, and she felt someone climb onto the mattress and crawl in next to her. It woke her up, or she dreamed she woke, because the mattress moved. She was lying on her stomach, and she lifted her head up and looked around groggily. There was no one there, and she relaxed and put her head back down, glad she didn't have to deal with anything. Then, as she drifted off, she felt someone caress her bottom and slide hands beneath her hips, moving her slightly. Her eyes popped open and she looked straight ahead at the headboard, unwilling to turn around. Whatever it was began opening her thighs.

This should have been alarming, but she felt very sleepy and warm. She drifted off somehow and only awoke again when the mattress started moving rhythmically against the headboard. Someone was on her and in her, having sex. It wasn't upsetting, it even felt good, but she looked at the headboard again and thought, "This can't be happening; there's no one here."

The sensations we're capable of in dreams are, in their own way, even more vivid than the sensations we experience in everyday life. In the cool light of day this woman was fairly sure this was just a dream, but the reality of the sensations and the false awakenings made it confusing. A few people are capable of really opening their eyes, looking around to make sure they aren't dreaming, seeing with their eyes, while their brain is still dreaming. In those brief moments they can see what is around them, but may also see the "reality" being created in their dream.

This dreamer had just gone off on her own after living with someone for a few years. She was lonely and craving contact and sex. It's likely this dream represented a kind of sexual memory being played, while also incorporating her feelings about the fact that "there's no one there," in her bed or in her life at the moment.

Out-of-Body Experiences

They call them OOBEs, which stands for *out-of-body experiences*. They are the realistic sensation of slipping out of your body, maintaining your consciousness and a more subtle body. You are then free to fly around, visit places, and move through walls. They are more than just flying dreams, yet there are similarities. They are controversial, and many people dismiss them. Others become zealots, practicing and working on popping out of their bodies at will.

Most typically a person may have such an experience spontaneously once in a lifetime, and if you've had one you know they are real.

One woman reported she had her first OOBE after a night of particularly intense lovemaking with her partner. They had spent a long, very satisfying night together, and she felt all those orgasms had renewed every cell in her body, and even altered the climate in the room; the air was glowing. She drifted off to sleep, or assumed she was sleeping, when she felt she was floating, bobbing. She opened her eyes and saw only a blank texture in front of her. Then she realized it was the texture of the ceiling against which she was now floating.

She looked down at the bed and saw two people, herself and her partner. She tried to move through the ceiling, and stuck her arm through, but couldn't get her head and shoulders through. This was so odd. Surely she should just think where she wanted to go, and instead there seemed to be some trick to penetrating matter. "This can't be right," she thought, but looking down, there they were. Besides, she felt so lovely. No weight, so *breezy*. She swam through the air at first, like those movies of the astronauts practicing weightlessness. Finally she decided she wasn't going to waste this experience by getting stuck.

With that she slipped fluidly through the ceiling, up and out through the roof. The night was lovely, the stars were clear, and the moon was out. She stepped off the roof and slid into the sky, moving downward until she got a grip on her expectations. It was as if navigation were a matter of expectation and intention. She sailed around for quite a while and eventually found herself back in bed. When she got up the next day, she got a small stepladder and brought it into the bedroom, climbed up, and touched the texture of the ceiling. She is convinced this was not a dream.

Whether this was a dream or a metaphysical OOBE, this experience was almost certainly triggered by the closeness, pleasure, and energy of the night before. When love and sex are extraordinary, why should it surprise us if we fly clean out of our bodies one night?

One More Night

Most of us have fantasized about having just one more night in the arms of a lover. Sometimes it seems this hunger can conjure up a dream that things are as they once were, and for a brief time we soak up the happiness. Then when we awaken, we deal with the reality that is around us.

One woman told me that when her husband was unexpectedly killed, the shock and grief she felt was terrible. On top of the pain of losing him, there was a pervasive sense of unreality. It simply wasn't the way her life was supposed to go. They were just in the beginning of building their life together. Now the whole world didn't make sense; and she was amazed how nothing seemed solid anymore. What she didn't expect, though, was that her views about life were going to change even more.

One night, after crying herself to sleep as she did so often, she heard footsteps in the house. These were not just any footsteps; these were the sounds of her husband coming home. He was tossing his boots in the mudroom, his coat on the rack in the hall. She sat up in bed and hugged her knees. She glanced at the clock and saw she hadn't even fallen asleep yet; it was early. She called his name. There were no further sounds, but she felt him coming into the room, felt the mattress move as he sat down. She couldn't see him, but his presence was so real that she talked to him in case this wasn't a dream.

In the morning when she woke, the first thought she had was that her husband had *really* been there. She knew this might be desperation on her part, but even factoring that in, she couldn't deny the sensation that it had been real. Not only had the experience felt real and unlike a dream, but also, stunningly, she had the sense of his company. She was not upset that morning. Her heart felt a tiny bit lighter. She had had dreams before that he was not dead; it had all been a terrible mix-up. But when she awoke from those dreams she burst into tears, tortured by the tricks of the night. But that morning she was excited and touched.

In the next few weeks nothing unusual happened, but she carried with her a growing certainty that her husband was sometimes with her. It was just little things, coincidences, or the sensation of someone being in the room. One night, as she lay in bed about to fall asleep, she felt some weight beside her. Then she felt her husband slide next to her and wrap his arms around her.

Another night when she was sure she was indeed asleep, she felt her husband trying to pry her knees apart, then a breeze seemed to be blowing between her legs. She sat up in bed and scolded her husband. This was just getting a little too weird. It was wonderful that he was still alive wherever he was, but she really wasn't up to any kind of after-death sex scene.

After that, there were no more sexual overtures, and with time the visits became less frequent. She remains convinced that her husband really did come to visit her, and I have heard similar stories from others. If we were motivated to dismiss the felt-sense of what is real, we could argue that the bereaved are traumatized, not thinking clearly, and prone to illusions. Even so, most people have a pretty good handle on what really happened to them, particularly in retrospect. I am not sure that we ever could, or should, have sex with the dead, but I do believe that love is a connection that survives even death.

Sex in an Alternate Dimension

One woman who was separated from her partner dreamed that they met in an alternate dimension, like Heaven, to walk and talk. This dimension was like paradise, with trees, flowers, and water running through a beautiful city. They walked hand in hand. Instead of being defensive and awkward, he was warm and secure, looking deeply into her eyes as she spoke. He told her how much he loved her, and how nothing that happened or failed to happen between them mattered in the larger sense.

She was relieved and felt close again. She put her arms around him. As they embraced, he kissed her and with the kiss she was drawn into the place where he was standing and he was drawn into her. They became a single column of light, vibrating and suspended as they merged. This was a kind of sex, comparable to but very different from sex on earth. It was sheer electricity. With a flash there was a kind of climax more intense than an orgasm. She stepped back and laughed, shaken. Some of him was still inside her, and some of her was inside him. They had exchanged some of their current.

When she awoke from this dream, she hoped that might mean they could work things out. But when they met a week later to have one of those stiff breaking-up dinners, she found that nothing had changed. Though they cared for each other, neither of them wanted this relationship at this time. Why then had the dream been so extraordinarily real? One possibility is that they did have a meeting in some other space and time, where they could sort things out at the level of their souls, exchanging a gift of energy that would be with them always.

She came away feeling that love is never wasted. In a paradoxical way, the experience in the dream gave her a sense of being close to him and also of being suddenly more able to let go. It certainly seems that for her, this dream helped her to find closure without as much sadness.

Dreaming in Tandem

There is an interesting body of work being done now on a phenomenon called *mutual dreaming*. It is also sometimes called shared dreaming. Essentially it is the experience of dreaming the same thing as your friend, roommate, lover, or family member. One person begins to share last night's dream at the breakfast table, and the other person bursts into tell the rest of the dream because they had the same dream! There are degrees of the experience; sometimes the entire dream is shared verbatim, sometimes people have essentially the same experience, like meeting friends near the Grand Canyon. Opinions differ on how useful this experience may be, and how, if we can cultivate it, should we use it? Some siblings share recurring dreams, reporting that sometimes they have it together and sometimes they just have "that same dream," almost as if they checked out a DVD.

I began having a version of mutual dreaming about a decade ago. I dreamed of teaching a class with local dream enthusiasts and went on a tangent about some facet of dream work. The next day I ran into one of the students who had been in my dream "class" the night before. The first thing out of her mouth was that she had just had a dream about me the night before in which she had attended a class I was teaching. She then said I had been explaining a rather intricate theory in her dream. (Evidently I'm just a huge blabbermouth, even when asleep.) We compared notes and found that we had pretty much been in the same place. After half a dozen incidents like this, I began to suspect that somehow our dreams do sometimes overlap.

A few years later a different layer of mutual dreaming started to emerge spontaneously. A friend I was close to was struggling with a relationship that had some real highs and lows. She's spunky and smart and wanted to give it a real try. Sometimes as I was dreaming at night, she would just walk into the landscape of my dream like an actor barging through the backdrop of a scene. She'd say: "Oh, sorry. I'm having a dream right now about Joe, and I wondered if I could get your take on something . . ." Then she'd tell me how the dream went, what she thought of it so far, and how she wanted to get to the heart of the matter.

She appeared to be having lucid dreams to try and work out the relationship, and then it would occur to her to pop over to me to get my view. This happened so often that I finally asked her to knock it off. There's nothing worse than butting into a friend's relationship under the umbrella of psychology, even if you're both dreaming at the time. She didn't remember these experiences when awake, but in every case, she didn't just appear in my dream as a character, she popped in from her own dream-in-progress next door. I felt some growing change coming from that quarter. The relationship? She finally drew her conclusions and ended it. Shortly after that, she met the man who was to become her husband and has never looked back. Whatever she did in those lucid-process dreams, she was on to something.

Dream Key #18

What Is Your PSI Quotient?

Some of us are more prone than others to unusual experiences. Just as some people are sensitive, musical, or funny, others are tuned in to intuitive and psychic experiences. It's wise to be cautious and pragmatic about these things without placing too much weight on them. My suspicion is that just as there are good thoughts and stupid ideas, so there are also valuable psychic moments, and junk-food psychic moments. Just because something comes through a nonlocal channel doesn't make it profound or spiritual. Always ask yourself if something is kind or wise and trust your own truth detector more than anyone else's. If you are prone to these moments, it will help you to accept that fact and don't get in a flap when something comes up. Take a look at the statements below and see how many of them ring true to your experience.

1. You sometimes know who is on the phone before you pick it up.

2. You take immediate likes and dislikes toward places and people.

3. You have had dreams that came true.

4. Someone in your family is known to be psychic.

5. You sometimes get a feeling of dread before something bad happens.

6. You sometimes imagine that you can read minds, hearing what people are thinking.

7. You can almost hear your pets talking to you in your mind.

8. Sometimes you have heard words or phrases pop into your mind when you were thinking about something entirely different.

9. You have lots of coincidences in your life.

10. There is one area in your life where you trust your intuition absolutely.

11. You have déjà vu experiences fairly often.

12. When you have something on your mind, the radio or television will coincidentally have a program or play a song that is right on point.

13. Sometimes you can just do something well, even though you have no idea how it's supposed to go, and have never done it before.

14. When you walk into a room and pets are present, they will usually look up and look you right in the eye, as if they know you.

If you recognized yourself in many of the above statements, you may be inclined to extraordinary experiences. Think of this as a trait, not a value system. It has little to do with whether you think it's possible, and it has nothing to do with your religion. If you have a psychic knack, accept that and use it as wisely as you can, just as you would any of your intelligences or abilities.

CHAPTER NINETEEN

Soul Mates

Anyone who works with dreams is familiar with questions on the suitability of partners, specifically: can our dreams help us find a soul mate, and can our dreams tell us whether the person in our sights is "the one"? As you already know, it's very possible to have great chemistry and a great time with someone who will leave your life a shambles. So this is tricky territory. While dreams may be hard to interpret on the surface, they tend to be strictly honest in their assessment of potential partners and adventures.

Dreams can tell us about sexual chemistry ahead of time, and they seem to know when we're at an intersection where a relationship is going to crop up. I am not sure whether we get ripe for a relationship, we dream of having one and then we create one, or whether our dreams race ahead in time somehow, sniff the wind, and weave a story about the relationship on the horizon. For women, at least, I often see that dreams will heat up, and then we'll suddenly find ourselves in a relationship. Perhaps this is a kind of sex therapy, keeping us connected with our feelings and our fantasies so that when we make a good connection, our systems and our feelings are tuned up.

The Best Sex

One woman was going around with a male friend who was very gentlemanly and courtly, almost like he'd stepped out of an old movie. They didn't know each other well, but they seemed to like the same things and he treated her with charming courtesy. After a little while she started to think that he might be gay, or at least bisexual, because there was nothing physical going on between them. She wasn't quite sure what to make of their friendship, but it was gentle and relaxing not to feel any pressing agenda. One night she had a stunning dream that she was having sex with her friend, and it was the best sex of her life. He was something else, and their chemistry lit up the sky. She scratched her head over that one, but it made her wonder. Eventually, a few months later, they started to have a physical relationship, and sure enough, it was incredibly exciting and satisfying. Their relationship wasn't a lifetime connection, but it was a case where her dreaming mind picked up on something that she would never have consciously considered: that she had some *really* nice nights ahead of her.

Dreams of Destiny Markers

There are moments we seem fated to encounter. People we are meant to meet, times when we can make a difference or when someone is there to help us. I don't feel that everything is already laid out in some fatalistic roadmap of life, but there do seem to be *destiny points* of special significance that are simply meant to be. The rest of the adventure is a matter of choice, creativity, luck, and intention. I think that fate puts some lights on the runway and that's it. The take-off, flight plan, and landing are up to us.

When we come to an intersection with fate, it is almost inevitably marked and acknowledged in our dreams.

One woman had a series of dreams in which a man and a woman, unknown to her, would travel toward each other, meet, and have a love affair. The people were different in each dream, and always fictional, unknown to her. Only the theme was constant: Two people were traveling, often great distances and through hardships to be together. After two months of these dreams, she suddenly met a man who struck a cord with her that she had never known before, and they embarked on a relationship that lasted many years. I have heard this type of story a number of times from women. That dreams seemed to foretell an important relationship, although in a vague way, as if noting changes in the climate or predicting a change in the seasons.

The Arms of an Angel

One woman had a very sweet dream that a celebrated colleague whom she admired very much was also an angel. He was both human and angel. During a time when she was very beleaguered with worries and frustrations, she dreamed that she spent the night in his arms. Somehow it felt perfectly natural that she should be having sex with an angel. It was both sexy and reassuring to look up into the canopy made by his wings. In the morning, and for some time thereafter, she felt infused with strength and hope.

This man was not someone she had ever had a relationship with in waking life, except as the most generally acquainted colleagues. But she knew his story and had always felt a kind of soul-connection with him. In another time, or another lifetime, who knows? She isn't pining away for this man, nor does she typically think of him in any sexual way. But since the dream, she has felt oddly encouraged to strike out in a new direction with her career. Somehow the dream-night in his arms was like a kind of endorsement, a stamp of approval and encouragement from the universe. Now, in the real world this doesn't add up. But it happens this way all the time. You can't do something on Tuesday, you have a dream that pours some kind of love into you, and on Wednesday you have a new strength and something previously impossible becomes doable.

The Difference Between Soul Mates and Destiny Markers

Some people are in our lives as nudges. There is something almost spooky about them. We love them fully and forever at short notice, even though we will never have a relationship with them and may not want one. It's like *ka-boom*: That sound you hear as you meet them is the sound of your heart flopping open like a garage door. You may feel like you already know them, or they understand you more deeply. You *may* feel you want to put them in your pocket or eat them with a spoon, because this kind of familiar-squishy recognition is pretty attractive. When I speak with women over forty, they say that earlier in life they didn't realize how accurate these feelings were. Over time the people that we feel this mystery-love thing with really are important to us; they have some purpose or meaning in our lives. But rather than project a love story onto the screen, we might do better to listen to the messages in our dreams to find out what kind of steps destiny is inviting us to dance.

The Big One

I know a woman who used to attract partners who needed a lot of help. She would calm down the nervous, dry out the drunk, and civilize the barbarians. Then, when she was exhausted and the guys were pretty spiffed up, the relationship would evaporate, and the man would enthusiastically leave, thanking her for enabling him to qualify for the really nifty partner he was now enjoying.

At one point she sort of bottomed-out with the pattern. A man she thought was the big one quit smoking, reunited with his estranged children, quit being so compulsive, and learned to take time away from work. Then the relationship hit the skids. They parted abruptly, and she grieved a great deal. One of the things she missed most was their sex life, which had been pretty great. She tossed and turned at night, alternating between sadness and frustration.

One night, like a gift, she had a dream that he had come

back into her bedroom for one last night. Every point on her body seemed to rise up and salute him as *the man*, and they fit together hungrily. When they slowed down a bit, she asked him if he would stay, since they were surely soul mates. He looked at her and smiled, and said, "You've got to stop trying to turn every aching heart on earth into your soul mate."

When she woke up, it was as if this fellow had kissed her goodbye in the night and helped set her free from her pattern. She had not given much thought to the idea that somewhere deep inside she felt she had to earn love by fixing something. But that was part of what kept her in the cycle, even when she no longer wanted to repeat it. Whatever the source of the change, she seems to have kicked her own habit, and is in a long-term relationship that seems to be going strong and requiring no major overhauls.

Dream Key #19
Soul-Searching

The first thing every woman wonders about when she has a sexual dream is, what it implies for her love life. If you're single you wonder if the dry spell is over, if you're with someone, you wonder if you should tactfully, playfully, bring up some of the highlights to your partner. The answer is probably yes on both counts. If you have a really sexy dream, you're more likely to be receptive to and thinking about getting close to someone in the near future. (However, don't go home with some scary weirdo the next night because you think your dream told you to!)

If you're with someone, if you can tactfully bring up some of the excitement you felt in your dream to your partner, it is likely your tale will be met with reasonable goodwill and attention.

1. Remember, you can be connected with someone on many levels, even spiritual levels, and it doesn't necessarily follow that you have to make a life together or even have a love affair. Soulfulness isn't the same thing as compatibility or destiny.

2. Sometimes dreams of soul connections are trying to nudge us to make some change or address something important. Honor the destiny markers in your dreams and don't try to force an interpretation on them. Let them speak to you.

3. If you're getting intoxicating signals in your dreams, get ready for some passionate phase to open up in your life. It may be a relationship, but it may also be about doing work that sets your soul on fire, or finding something you were truly born to experience.

4. It's a delicate balance, being willing to dance with fate and honor the mysterious timing of our lives, yet not be too passive or goofy about it all. Since your dreams are in tune with this subtle pulse of life, keep an eye on them to let you know when the season of passion is upon you.

CHAPTER TWENTY

Intimate Intuition: The Rating Game

One of the most valuable attributes of dreams is their ability to express subtle insights overlooked by ordinary consciousness. Intuitive leaps can save time, and in some cases provide early warning as if by recognizing patterns instantly. The dreaming mind appears to be intent on creating and preserving positive relationships, as if operating from an instinct to protect the dreamer. In terms of providing information that can be useful, erotic dreams are high-value products of the mind. Many dreams that express sexuality or explore relationships appear to combine the best of three psychological strengths.

Dream Vigilance is the tendency of the mind to scan for threat and to amplify that threat in dreams, presumably so that if we register what is going on we can respond to it effectively.

The Relationship Imperative is the mind's preoccupation with community, family, and connectedness. Women dream more often about love, relationship, friendship, and community than anything else. By day we may work like dogs, scurrying to our meetings, but by night, the dreaming mind is like an intrusive aunt, saying: "Darling, have you met anyone yet? What about that boy you used to go around with, whatever happened to him?" Regardless of what we claim to want or expect, our dreams are sticking with the notion that love, sex, and connection form the staff of life. In other words, dreams have a bias, and that bias is *toward* a relationship; with yourself, a significant other, family, extended family, and spirit. The agenda of the dreaming mind is, at least in part, to get you connected and keep you connected with love.

Intimate Intuition is the lightning-like ability of the unconscious mind to recognize patterns with minimal data. When you meet someone and make a potentially intimate contact, your intuition does immediate cross-referencing against past experiences including your subliminal reactions to the person in question. Your dreams then extrapolate about the future, often providing the equivalent of a thumbs-up or thumbs-down.

Jean-Claude Van Damme and the Rotten Molar

A lovely woman was having a fling with a fellow whom she knew was not right for her. He seemed unkind to her pets, intolerant of her children, and sarcastic with her. However, he was good in bed, wealthy, and took her traveling with him to places she enjoyed. She was trying to enjoy herself for the time being and keep the negative things at bay.

One night she had a dream of having great sex with the action star Jean-Claude Van Damme. He was so flexible and strong, and she loved his chiseled features. But after the sex, he got up and went to the bathroom, and she felt something funny in the back of her mouth. She rolled her tongue around and felt a loose molar. She probed it with her tongue, and it lifted up from her gum sickeningly. She was able to spit it into her hand and taste a little blood in her mouth.

When something nasty is juxtaposed right in the middle of an otherwise positive sexual dream, it's time to make note of it. This is the psyche trying to tell you there's a cockroach in your soup; that you need to pause and look closely before you proceed. Blood loss in dreams is usually associated with a subjective loss of power or energy, and damage to teeth is frequently a signal that something is eroding the dreamer's autonomy. This dream was deliberately stitching together the things that she kept separate in her mind by day: the fun sexual excursions with the side effects of being with someone who was not really good for her. When she finally broke things off with him, he was harder to get rid of than she had expected, and things got somewhat nasty, although not violently so.

Still, it was very much as if her dreaming mind had issued a warning that turned out later to be accurate. In a twist of fate, in the month after getting out of this arrangement, she met a terrific man who would later become her husband. This is someone who is thrilled to be with her, loves animals, and has a great relationship with her kids. Had she still been playing with rotten-molar man, perhaps she would not have the life she has now. Dreams are constantly nudging us toward what will nourish us and make us happy, and they are trying to ease us away from the little mistakes and messes that occur.

Just as intimate intuition can provide a warning by putting a nasty image in the middle of a love scene, it can also mark the potential for joy by placing images of fulfillment around the setting of an erotic interlude.

Corn-Fed Love

There was a woman who was dating a fellow who was almost too nice. He was the sort who had everything going for him except sizzle. She was impressed with him mentally, ticking off his good qualities, but wasn't sure about their physical and emotional compatibility, at least at first.

Just as their relationship was getting closer, she had a dream that made her take a second look. In the dream they were walking hand in hand through a cornfield, looking for a place to throw down a blanket and make love. The rows were tall, and the couple disappeared together into what felt like another world. Finally they found a place deep in the heart of the cornfield, and they lay down, quietly making love with only the sound of the corn rustling in the breeze around them. She felt hot and lazy and peaceful. She had often associated sex with feeling rushed, hungry, and wanting to be filled. But there, in the corn, she felt that everything that mattered in the world was right there. Afterward, they got up and roamed around a quiet road nearby. He said he was taking her to a house he wanted her to see. They came to a nice country-style house and he said, "Here, this is the house where Mary lives; I wanted you to see it."

The images in this dream stayed with her, as did the tone. Corn, like other images of harvest, is a symbol of fertile possibilities, success, and positive cycles. It is interesting that this dream gave her a sexual tryst in the midst of a very robust cornfield, as if to say, "Don't miss this opportunity; everything you've ever wanted is right here." The dream also went to further lengths to provide a hint when he took her to look at the house where Mary lives. Often in dreams houses are really mental frameworks or ideas. In a symbolic way the dream was saying: This is a place in your life when you might marry. The chance, the person, and the timing are right here, take a good look at it.

She did take a look and realized that this relationship really was what she wanted, it simply had come in a form that she wasn't expecting, so she had almost overlooked it. Dreams that have a touch of intuition involved are often wiser than we are at recognizing the difference between form and essence. Sometimes what we want is nearer than we think, but we're searching so hard for the mental picture we have of happiness that we miss the real happiness that is right beside us.

Nice Ring, Where's the Diamond?

The objects in your dreams are often meaningful in symbolic terms. An engaged woman had a dream that she and her fiancé were trying to have sex in a hammock that kept turning over and dumping them on the ground. They kept climbing back in the hammock and trying different strategies. She got on top and straddled him, trying to balance with the tips of her toes touching the ground on either side. But as soon as she moved and lifted one toe, *flip*, they were on the ground again.

They repeated the process with him on top and went crashing in short order. While they were on the ground, she looked down at her hand to admire her engagement ring and noticed something she had never seen before. It really contained no diamond; the prongs contained a piece of striated metal cut to shine as if it were a stone. She thought that was weird and was disappointed, but didn't want to seem critical of it, so she didn't say anything. Her fiancé was talking about how they should get back in the hammock and lie facing each other on their sides this time. She stared at her ring, distracted, and wondered how she might suggest they just go into the house and get on the bed.

It's human nature to take something that isn't working and to just doggedly keep doing it, as if we're going to one day get a new and successful result. Dreams turn the spotlight on this pattern by creating crazy tasks we struggle with like stooges from an old movie: typically making matters worse and wearing ourselves out. In this dream the diamond represents the whole package; the love, the life, the marriage, and the future. She has gotten into the habit of glancing at her ring in waking life, and the habit carried through into the dream. Yet in the dream she notices something she has not seen before, there is no stone here. There is only a simulated piece of metal that catches the light. In addition, the dream places them in what appears to be a ludicrous situation. They want to have sex, but the hammock keeps dumping them.

Many erotic dreams turn to frustration themes as the characters struggle to find the right place or the right opportunity for sex. The struggle for place, privacy, and proximity are really metaphors for the struggles to "find the love" or "find the sizzle" in our connections. When we can't get it right in our dreams, we often cannot get it right in the relationship, either.

This woman was struck by the dream and its implications.

She was gradually feeling disenchanted with her fiancé, yet was on the marriage express and the train had already gathered a great deal of momentum. The thought of creating a fuss and spoiling the story line at that point was too appalling, and so they moved forward. With luck they will find their way with fewer bumps in the future. At the very least, she knows her dreams can be a source of insight if she ever feels the need for another perspective.

Not You Again!

One of the most critical favors our dreams can do for us is to give us a quick reading on our new connections. The dreams you have after meeting someone, starting a relationship, or making a decision are often commentaries on the wisdom of the decision and are often stunningly accurate predictors of the future.

A woman who was dating a very charming person was naturally excited and having fun with him. But the same week they started seeing a lot of each other, she had a dream about an important disappointment in her past. In the dream she was back with her ex-lover, and they were having sex. Physically the sex was okay, but she kept staring at his greasy hair and thinking numbly: "What have I done? Why am I back with him again? He is the king of jerks!" It was very depressing, and she couldn't understand in the dream how they had wound up together again.

She knew the dream was something of a cautionary note, but when she explored it, she kept thinking new Mr. Smoothie is nothing like old Mr. Jerk. Indeed, they were dramatically different in appearance and style. But remember, dreams detect essence or core, the way a metal detector finds gold. Her dream meter was going off at the "jerk" marker, and the best emblem for that in her storage base of memories was the poster boy for disappointment in her past. While the conscious mind is busy rationalizing and being captivated, the dreaming mind will instantly alert and say, *Oh, going back to the poison trough one more time, are we?*

Fortunately, her dreams kept battering away at the gate of her consciousness, while the smoothie began to show he was a little too smooth. They parted company, and she emerged unscathed, later discovering that he had an alarming history and that she had gotten off easily compared to some of his contacts.

Dream Key #20

Making the Most of Intuitive Erotic Dreams

Sexual, erotic, and relationship dreams are usually "in you face," because the psyche is determined you will be loved and connected in this life. Here are four things to look for in your dreams to see if they may include intimate intuitions about your connections and what will make you happy.

1. Is the **setting** in the dream one that works? Dreary, crowded, sinking, or confusing settings are signals that something is "off" in your personal life. Lovely settings, with open space, privacy, or good vibrations, are usually a positive sign that you're on the right track.

2. Are the **objects** in the dream functional and positive? Broken objects, leaky plumbing, sinking ships, and empty rings are warnings that you may not be nourished by what is going on. Things that work well, or which fit your desires and heart perfectly, are often signs that your current situation is positive and right for you.

3. If **people** from the past crop up, are they people who treated you well? If you think of people from the past as commemorative stamps, what quality or emotion would they commemorate?

4. The **timing** of a dream is critical. If you are making an important decision, or are hooking up or falling for someone, pay attention to the reading your dreaming mind gives on the situation. Paying attention to your intimate intuition is just another way of playing it smart and being true to your heart and your passions.

PART FIVE

Accepting Your Power and Passion

CHAPTER TWENTY-ONE

Rescue Themes

Many women report dreams involving themes of rescue. Movies and books offer us recurring images of women being rescued by brave souls who later become lovers. Yet in dreams, it is often the women who perform the rescue, saving lost people from oblivion or death. Not all these dreams include scenes of sex, but in many of them it is understood that the person being saved from exile is a sexual partner or soon will be.

As you read these descriptions, remember that dreams tell physical stories about feelings and qualities. If they did not, we presumably would just dream about blobs floating around colliding with one another. Sometimes the prisoners of war or the wrongly convicted felons are images of something in life that has been shut off or put aside. If you have such a dream while you are in a relationship, it may certainly have something to do with your partner, some quality that is being redeemed through your connection. But it you have a dream like this when you are single, chances are greater that the story may have something to do with a side of yourself associated with passion that has been kept at bay for some time.

The Artists' Prison Colony

Artistic souls have a tough time in our society. They can't seem to rest or feel alive unless they are somehow expressing their talent, but they are under lifelong pressure to do something non-arty and to discard their interests to play the odds of success.

The tendency to polarize our complex qualities is pervasive. As I mentioned before, with respect to our sexual identities we tend to think of ourselves as either hot nymphomaniacs or neutered robots. In a similar fashion, artists report they feel great pressure to either make it big as an artist or never have anything to do with art. That doesn't leave much room for the spontaneous quality of their gifts.

If the only two choices in life are miraculously becoming an artistic superstar, or abandoning your gifts forever, what choice do you functionally have? Most people uneasily abandon their gifts to earn a living, as if there were a law against continuing to express them once you get a job. The promise is that one day, maybe if there is enough time and money, you will pull out the art from your storage unit and have "earned" the right to explore it. This all-or-nothing perspective is one of the ways we drive ourselves crazy and starve ourselves for the passions that can nourish us most.

One woman had a dream that she had come in contact with an artist who was serving a prison sentence in a colony of art prisoners. This was hazily in some foreign land where it was illegal to be artistic, and those people who had created works of art were imprisoned for it. She did not dare tell anyone she was an artist herself, for fear she might be imprisoned, too. But she determined to see if she might take steps to get her friend out of the encampment. She went to visit him and saw what these artists did all day, carrying burdens to and fro for the guards, injuring their hands on nails and wire that stuck out from the boxes they moved around.

One of the emaciated artists could not get a good grip on a box and almost dropped it. The guards quickly nailed his hands to the burden so that there would be no more slipping.

The woman dashed away and held a series of meetings to get her friend released. She visited places like Amnesty International and the United Nations, searching for some loophole through which he might be released. Then they found an obscure law that if a woman claimed one of the convicts and would marry him and take responsibility for him, he would be released and she could take him home. This is what she did. The prisoner was turned over to her, and she took him home, nursing him back to health. He was haggard and starved, and there were many wounds that she washed and bandaged. As they sat together and drank tea at her kitchen table, he put a bandaged hand over hers and a charge of heat moved through her right into her heart.

Rescue dreams are memorable and have very consistent movielike plots. Everything revolves around the injustice and horror of the person in exile, while the dreamer desperately tries to find the means to save the person. It is not difficult to suspect since the dreamer is an artist that the imprisoned artists represent the side of her nature that feels beaten down and criminal for what she loves. In this land, it is illegal to create art. Presumably one can *be* an artist with some im-punity, as long as one does not actually *create* anything. Notice the very specific detail the dream presents about the injury and torture of the hands. These artists are actually nailed to their nonartistic burdens in a way that is subtly a crucifixion. This lets us get a taste of the subjective pain of the artistic spirit that is unable to be what it is. They are kept from creating, and they are forced to just move boxes around all day.

Yet this dream suggests this particular artist is struggling to shake off the spell of polarization. There must be some way to get this guy out of that hellhole, and she is going to find it. As nasty as some of the hardships in our dreams may be, they are made worthwhile by the solutions they often present. The way to break the spell, to release the imprisoned artist, is to *marry him*. In the language of dreams, marriage, like sex, is symbolic of uniting, embracing, and connecting. What she needs to do, and what she presumably is doing, is to lick her wounds and bring this part of herself into her life more, to create a partner-ship with it.

What our inner aspects want is a chance to live and breathe. Sides of you that are built to create or express or communicate want to do just that. When they are not allowed even to *exist* they feel only like a wound that is better not thought about. This is why they appear in our dreams, showing us the ravages of their exile. They are not about how we make a living; they are about how we feel alive. This is why, as they sit drinking tea, his touch shoots a hot bolt of promise right to her heart. If she will rescue him and heal him, he will bring her heart alive.

The Hitchhiker

In another fairly common theme of rescue, a woman comes in contact with a wanderer who is mysteriously familiar. They have not met before, but as she picks him up and gives him a ride, everything about him seems familiar as if he were an old lover who had changed a great deal over time.

She keeps looking at his features and feeling as if they have met before as she drives. Eventually, they stop to get something to eat, and after sharing a meal and conversation, he finally confronts her about it. "I can't believe you don't remember me," he says sadly. She feels a rush of recognition, but still can't quite make the connection. "I do, sort of. I remember your face . . ." "Maybe this will help you remember," he says, and pulls her to him and kisses her. She feels how well they fit together, and everything about him seems made for her. They continue to kiss in a body-mauling way, out of breath and falling into a nearby doorway. She smoothes his hair from his forehead and says they should get back in her car and go somewhere. "I'm not going anywhere with you," he says sadly. "I'll just be out here somewhere when you're ready." He pulls away and walks off, leaving her standing in the doorway. He is going back to wandering. The implication is that if she could really remember him, then they would be together. Since she can't, the deal is off, although there is some hope that the offer is on the table if she can figure it out.

This enigmatic dream might as well have a neon sign that reads: "Important message here." Yet, like many dreams, it takes some work to find out what the important message is all about. To the best of her assessment, the wanderer looked like a television star who had great popularity as a young man and then he sort of disappeared. He was someone who showed great early promise, then for whatever reason disappeared from public view.

The dreamer herself had toyed with the idea of going into politics when she was very young, but life had gathered momentum and carried her in another direction. Recently she has had time to do volunteer work and other public service activities. There is a pulse beating in her somewhere that she has not felt in years. In a way, it is like encountering an old love, feeling that recognition, desire, and effortless compatibility without being able to explain it. Because her talents have to do with leadership and "star" quality, she is all the more alienated from them. While she is not going to race out and run for office, she is courting the challenge thrown out by the apparent nomad: She will try to *remember*, and perhaps he has something to teach her.

Edward Scissorhands

In the movie *Edward Scissorhands* the hero is a young man with a deformity: His hands are blades. He begins life all scarred up and isolated, then goes through a time of glory as it is discovered that he can cut hair, trim hedges, and make really great ice sculptures. This movie struck a chord with one woman, who dreamed she was involved with the main character in a dicey but ultimately fulfilling encounter.

In the dream the woman was trying to have sex with Edward Scissorhands. It was a perilous proposition because of course the least little touch with those hands would slice her to bits. At first they began with him on top of her, but as he propped himself up to get some leverage, his blades dangled horrifyingly in front of her face. In a way, it was hot being pinned helplessly beneath him and not being able to move one tiny bit. But it soon became clear that if he forgot himself even for a moment, she would be badly slashed. They stopped, and he carefully withdrew and moved off her. They got reorganized with him on his back, his blade-hands carefully extended out and away from her so she could be on top. This was much more satisfactory. She told herself that in this relationship, positioning was all-important.

This dream is somewhat typical of themes in which women explore sex with creatures that are not entirely human, or who might even be considered monsters. When they awaken, it is surprising that anyone would dream of sex with such a partner, but in the dreams, the sexual feelings flow and the attraction is just as overwhelming as under more normal circumstances. Edward Scissorhands is both a "star" and a victim of his deformity; it defines his life, and he can't get away from it. Everything he touches is "sculpted" and changed because of this quality. He cannot even pick something up without slicing it.

The dreamer is a woman with an extraordinary mind: like a laser beam or a scalpel. She is one of those people everyone admires, but they also hope she doesn't start to analyze their casually mentioned problems with her fierce logic. If she turns her attention to something, it is filleted in short order. While this is predominantly positive in her life, creating success and respect, it also has a shadow side. Some people are wary of her and find her judgmental, and sometimes after a meeting or conversation, she wonders in retrospect why she had to make mincemeat of someone's opinion or challenge every assumption she found faulty. We all have strengths that have become our primary modes of being in the world, and we tend to reach for them reflexively like old gunfighters at every encounter. Regardless of what the situation calls for, or the myriad ways we might respond, we usually pull out our favorite reflexive mode and then wonder afterward: "Why do I keep *doing* that?"

Dreams are deft at illustrating these dilemmas, and sometimes of offering clues as to how we can shift things around. In this dream the woman starts out entirely immobilized by the blades that seem to surround her. One possibility suggested is that she change her position. After all, the razorlike side of her is just one part, however important, of a larger personality. She can enjoy it without being paralyzed by it. The implication here is to identify with the larger self, to get on top of her intellect by identifying with her humanity first. She is a person with a gift, not a person possessed by her gift. This may sound abstract, but the way we channel and divide our energy, and the qualities in ourselves that we promote or imprison are a big deal to the unconscious mind.

Dream Key #21

Start Your Own Amnesty Program

Many rescue themes are intrapsychic. These dramas are metaphors for bringing submerged qualities into the light of day. Accepting your body, breaking the taboo against creating art, or following the path that called to you earlier in life. For a moment, think about your history, the things people told you were talents, or the things you loved. Look at the list below and consider aspects of personality or spirit that you suspect may have been locked in the attic for whatever reason.

Leadership ability
Star quality
Artistic ability
Communication skills
Writing
Being sexy
Being spiritual
Being a wise woman
Loving nature
Being creative
Being smart
Being of service
Bringing people together
Being powerful
Being in charge
Having needs of your own
Being able to articulate your needs
Honoring your nature
Having a personal rhythm
Being complex, paradoxical
Being more than your roles, job, and relationships

You probably have some things swimming around in your mind now that may not be listed above. Jot them down so you don't lose track of them. Think the forbidden thoughts.

. . .

Remember the tendency; call it a cultural trance, to view interests and gifts as all-or-nothing propositions. Start paying attention to the times when you feel pulled toward something, and then remind yourself to step away from it, because you won't be good enough at it, or it won't make money, or because you aren't the creative one in the family. We don't have to get carried away feeling we have to reform ourselves. It is simply that if we are awake in our own lives, then we have the freedom to change when it suits us, instead of staying on autopilot and wondering why we keep doing the same things.

CHAPTER TWENTY-TWO

Animals in Erotic Themes

Most sex dreams are easy to identify for obvious reasons. Other dreams explore the needs and hungers of erotic rhythms, but are less easy to identify on the surface. While women do not seem to dream of having sex *with* animals, we do often have animals within dreams that are dealing with sexual matters.

There's a Squirrel in My Pants

One woman dreamed that somehow a little squirrel had run up the inside of her pant-leg and had lodged itself in her crotch. She was shocked by this and wanted to run to get some help, but the squirrel tickled her every time she tried to move. It was horrible, but there was something arousing about the tickling. She was getting flushed and starting to get off on the sensations, God help her. She had to get that little sucker *out* of there. She was laughing, gasping, screaming, and flailing her arms.

At this point a handsome passerby saw her and came over to see what was going on. It was a television character named Grissom, from the TV show *CSI*. Between gasps and involuntary movements, she told him what had happened. He seemed to know just what to do, as if he rescued innocent women from sex-crazed squirrels every day. "Hold still," he said briskly, and shoved his hand down the front of her pants. She groaned, closed her eyes, and held still. Surely this situation was going to get even more humiliating if she didn't concentrate on not being aroused.

Just as quickly Grissom extracted the squirrel and sprang back with it in his hand. He moved away and tossed it into some nearby shrubs. She thanked him and tried to recover some shred of dignity. He was casual about the incident and seemed not to take in her flushed face. He gave her one of those happy-to-have-been-of-help-ma'am comments and they parted company.

The television character that appeared in her dream represented an ideal partner for this woman. Cool and competent, but also compassionate and sexy. She was not with anyone at the time of this dream, but was reviewing her history and thinking perhaps next time around she might try a different sort of person and a different sort of relationship. Although she would not describe her former lovers as "squirrelly," she had no doubt that the rodent that scurried into her drawers was probably representing the kind of accidental connections she has often had in the past. She would fall into a relationship, and stay in it because of the sex, getting "tickled" every time she considered making a move.

Interestingly, her ideal partner comes by in this dream to rid her of squirrel-sex once and for all. If nothing else, this gives her hope that being more purposeful in her choices in the future may be the right strategy for this time in her life.

The Giant Spider

Women dream about spiders a lot. There are a number of interpretations about what spiders represent. They are charged symbols that appear to mean different things in different sorts of dreams. In some cases, spiders represent the negative charge of sexuality: the dark, creepy, hurtful things that get mixed up in our sex drives and emotions.

One woman dreamed that she was in bed with her fiancé, and as they lay side by side sleeping, she felt something crawling on her. It moved, whispery soft, up her foot and leg. As she opened her eyes, she saw it was a hairy black spider as big as her hand. Her legs were slightly parted, and she knew that the spider was going to move upward and try to crawl inside her. She tried to wake up her fiancé by yelling, but her throat was somehow paralyzed, no words would come out. She tried to recoil from the spider, but she couldn't move. She lay there in a silent scream that came out only as a tiny croak.

Just then however, she heard someone calling her name. In real life her fiancé, who really was next to her, had heard her agonized croaking and had known she was having a nightmare. He kept softly calling her name and comforting her until she awakened. For some reason this dream was terribly upsetting, and she cried a little as he held her. It meant a great deal to her that he had awakened her, as if he had sensed her need for him while she was trapped in her tormenting dream.

This woman had been in an abusive marriage years before, and had endured a variety of psychological, physical, and sexual torment. After extricating herself from the situation, she had been through therapy, learned a profession, and made a home for herself and her child. Eventually she felt settled and healed enough for a relationship, and she met a wonderful man. They got engaged and were eagerly looking forward to their future. She felt comfortable, safe, and loved with him. As her system settled into this sanctuary and new beginning, a deep layer of pain and fear sometimes rippled through her. Sometimes new love that is good still touches scar tissue from the past. Her dream was showing some negative sexual scars, like a shadow creeping out now that she felt strong enough and safe enough to handle it.

Her fiancé, as if part of the dream, awoke her from her nightmare and comforted her. Symbolically this can be viewed as suggesting he was the very person to help her break the spell of the past, day by day, night by night. They have been together for many years now, quite happily, and the shadows of the past seem to have faded and lost their power.

The Blowfish

Women do not seem to share many dreams involving oral sex, for whatever reason. It's difficult to know if we don't dream about it much, or if people are reluctant to talk about it.

One woman dreamed that she had a pet blowfish that would swell up very big and then nestle between her legs and perform oral sex. Perhaps because it was a fish, all squishy and slippery, this was amazingly satisfying.

In her real life she was in a relationship where apparently she performed oral sex, but her partner did not. Though she described this as "no big deal," her puffy little blowfish *did* seem to be notable for being "very big." In the symbolism of dreams, sometimes, big images are code for important issues. She felt this was not something they could talk about, but she thought she might be able to navigate some kind of improved conditions by sheer wiggling and positioning.

Choking on a Snake

A woman found herself working in close proximity with a former lover who had been controlling and snarly with her, but also rather sexy. Time had passed since their relationship, and she felt it would be fine to work with him. She was struggling to keep everything professional and to focus on the work, but there was a certain charge in the air, and she thought he was making excuses for them to spend time together.

She had a dream that she was trapped in a dark dungeon filled with snakes that were penetrating all parts of her body. She was most concerned by one that was choking her. It was shoved all the way down her throat, and she found she couldn't breath. Just as she felt she might pass out, the snake pulled out of her mouth just in time.

These snakes seem to serve dual symbolic duty: They are

obviously phallic and sexual, penetrating her as they are. They are also classic "trouble," which snakes also tend to represent.

This dream was essentially warning this woman that she was getting herself into a pickle. The sexual energy was getting so strong that she was practically choking on it. But the setting in the dungeon was like a neon sign reading: This way for loss of freedom!

She extricated herself from the work situation as quickly as was feasible and put distance between them.

The Mare and the Stallion

A friend of mine has a beautiful mare that is her pride and joy. The horse and rider are well suited as they are both spirited, tough, and adventurous. She boards the horse at a stable with riding trails and turnouts where the horses can visit and relax.

She dreamed that one day she went to the barn and found that a stallion had broken into the mare's turnout and had mated with her. She was initially indignant and angry. But as she went to check on the mare and see if she had been injured, she found the mare sweaty, happy, and glowing. She usually only had that look after a reckless gallop through the woods. Her mane was tangled, her eyes were soft, and she sighed with contentment. "Oh. I see," the woman said. "Finally she got some."

This dreamer is a newlywed. Her contentment with her spouse and their suitability for each other are obvious. She is an independent sort and the process of becoming a life partner has been gradual, but it's clearly a wonderful time in her life. This dream of her horse's "surprise sex," and subsequent contentment, likely parallels her own happiness and fulfillment at this time in her life.

Riding the Wild Horses

Horses are often associated with vitality and aliveness in dreams. Perhaps this is why many dreams seem to provide feedback about our health and vigor by images of horses that are either thriving or wasting away.

One woman was finally emerging from the low period following her divorce. It was necessary, evidently, and she and her kids would ultimately be better for the change. But it had taken a while to shake the doldrums of loneliness and to stop feeling that she had failed.

She knew she was on the road to recovery when she had a dream that she was riding a big black stallion bareback through the woods. Their every movement was perfectly balanced, and they soared over fallen logs and brush as if he might have wings. The pounding of his hooves and the wind through her hair were invigorating and sensual. She wrapped her legs tightly around him to stay on, but they moved as one unit through space.

At the time of this dream she had just met a slightly younger man who was interested in pursing her. She was flattered and unsure whether it would be a good idea to embark on some kind of connection when she just had the sense of the ground beneath her feet. On top of that, she was not feeling her most alluring after the divorce and becoming a single parent. The responsibility and "the mommy thing," seemed to have eaten her alive.

But this carefree, zesty little dream made her think that she wasn't "over the hill" just yet. It would be nice to have a fling, if nothing more, to let herself feel like a woman again. The fellow apparently proved to be not only worth trying out, but very taken with her indeed, and they have been together ever since.

Feed That Wildcat, Will You?

Just as horses can represent our vitality, cats sometimes are uniquely feminine in their symbolism. Dreams that feature harm coming to cats sometime imply wounding to the feminine spirit or sexuality.

A number of women have reported dreams of feral cats or wildcats. In these dreams the wildcat has often been neglected or starved. When an animal in a dream is suffering neglect, it is most likely an aspect of the dreamer that has been ignored or has not received much attention lately. If this is a dog, it may represent the playful, fun-loving, uncomplicated side of the dreamer. If the neglected animal is a cat or a special wildcat, the dream may be more sexual in nature.

A woman had a dream that she emerged onto the front porch of her house and discovered a wildcat that had been living there. She vaguely remembered the cat, it belonged to her, even though it was wild and would not come into the house. She looked down at it, and it twirled and purred as if begging for food. Then she realized that she had not actually *fed* this wildcat in five years. Wow. She rushed to get some food for it, feeling bad. How had she gotten distracted for five straight years and forgotten to take care of this thing?

This dreamer had recently met someone she liked very much and the sparks were flying. It was as if she were waking up after a very long sleep, and she was enjoying the process. This little "wildcat" was probably her own sensual nature that had been living on bread and water for quite some time.

None of us can have it all, in all chapters of our lives. But if you find yourself dreaming of an animal in need of care or rescue, see if you can interpret what the symbolism might be trying to say. Sometimes it is just time to feed the wildcat.

Dream Key #22

Finding the Gift in Dream Animals

Think of the animals, if any, that you have in your dreams. Are they robust and exciting or undernourished and shivering? Women shy away from identifying with animals that are powerful and wild, tending to think that big scary jaguar in the living room couldn't possibly mean anything, and certainly isn't a part of themselves. While dreamers themselves are the ultimate authority on what their dreams mean, sometimes we can benefit from a nudge to consider what an image might represent. Below is a list of qualities that animals represent in dreams. Refer to if when you have a puzzling dream image.

Vitality
Sexuality
Wildness
Power
Survival instincts

Familial instincts
Happiness and loyalty
Vulnerability
Wisdom
Shrewdness
Perspective

CHAPTER TWENTY-THREE

Complex Stories, Hot Sex

If our dreams are any indication, many of us have to go through a lot of strange shenanigans to have great sex. While there are dreams that involve a single glance followed by ripping clothes and gasping orgasms, more often than not women's erotic dreams are complicated.

Kissing Cousins

One woman has a cousin who had always given her the feeling that, if they weren't related, they might hook up somehow. Nothing untoward has ever passed between them, but their connection is so obvious that other family members and friends have cautioned her that it's a little funny. She would love to spend more time with him, but all things considered, they've both taken pains to keep everything nice and cousiny. One year, though, she went to a big family reunion and spent the night in a big campground with everyone else. She felt the same sort of bond with her cousin that she always does, and in keeping with their unspoken decision, they were friendly but kept a careful distance. That night, as she slept in her sleeping bag in her little tent, she had a dream that allowed her to have a forbidden adventure at the same time it satisfied all potential objections to the project.

In the dream her parents had told her at the reunion that she was now old enough to be told the truth: She was adopted. They had simply not wanted to upset her until now. Far from being upset by the news, she was overjoyed. Her family had never quite seemed right anyhow. She quickly found her cousin to tell him the good news. He was as pleased as she, and later slipped into the tent to congratulate her personally. Finally she got to run her hands over his tanned skin and kiss the mouth she knew so well. When he took off his pants, he seemed unusually well endowed and had a striking erection. She made some comment like, "Well, there, anyone could see we're not related," and they had a serious fit of giggling until they climbed into the sleeping bag.

When she awoke in the morning, the feeling of the sleeping bag around her felt sensual, as if the events of the night before, and her elaborate dream, were all real. Finally she'd gotten *that* out of her system. But she laughed at the great lengths her mind had gone to in getting her cousin out of his jeans. Her whole life history had to be rewritten so she could have a sexy dream. But the dream served a dual purpose. It was fun, it let her explore something taboo that was never going to happen in the real world, and it wrapped it up very playfully in a little joke so that this isn't a dark corner any-more, it's a cute sassy dream-memory and can be filed under "finished business."

Sometimes our dreams seem to use complexity to make it okay for us to try something, or someone, different. At other times elaborate scenarios serve to heighten the passion, lifting us outside our everyday thoughts so that we can be exclusively sensual for a time.

Vampire Initiation Party

One thing Anne Rice has done for contemporary culture is to make vampires sexy; they were suggestive before, but in the land of our dreams, these guys have really taken hold. Vampire dreams are not all fun or sexy, but those that seem like dream-fantasies are usually the dreams of women in their teens through thirties.

One young woman had a dream that she belonged to a group of people slowly being taken over by vampires. One by one, the vampires singled people out, sucking their blood and turning them into the undead. Everyone's fate seemed sealed, but then the head vampire saw her and made an alternative offer. If she would come to his party and have sex with him there in front of all the new vampires for as long as he wanted, then he would stop harvesting her friends and would let them all go. In the way of dreams, he happened to be a sexy fellow with a lot of presence, kind of scary, but only enough to make things interesting. Feeling hugely heroic, she agreed to the plan. Although she didn't let on to anyone, she might have gone for him anyway, because he had a powerful hypnotic quality that was like a drumbeat getting louder the longer she was in his presence.

There was some kind of circular stage in the middle of the party, and she saw that he wasn't kidding about doing it in front of everybody. That was a little awkward, because everybody got quiet and turned around to watch when he made her get up on it. But this drumbeat thing was still going on, and she felt increasingly dizzy, confused, and hot; it felt good to lie down. She noticed that she was naked, but then she was looking at the vampire and could feel but no longer see the staring faces all around them. She expected him to drop his cape, but he didn't, he just leaped up on the stage and onto her in a second. He wrapped his mouth around her throat and then pushed her legs apart. She felt her mind fluttering away like something in the distance, wondering if he was going to bite her or kill her. He pushed inside her and exacted his "price" for quite a long time, without any biting or violence. Presumably her friends got to go free, but we'll never know, because the sex got so good she forgot all about them and the dream just ended there.

For a dream about undead parasitic monsters, this is a pretty clean-cut and satisfying. This is almost a Disney sex vampire, with no nasty qualities. The plot is set so that she can take a walk on the wild side, but it's strictly for heroic reasons. This is a young woman who appears to be reveling in her sexual powers, and possibly is somewhat awed by how potent attraction and seduction can be. (The whole sexual act is up on a pedestal in a sense.) She gets to practice exhibitionism, but only for a good cause. She gets to feel like a sexual knockout, because the vampire saw her and had to have her. She has sex with a monster, but he's a good lover who apparently just wants straight sex and doesn't even bite her.

The actions of this dream vampire add to the piquancy and permission to be swept away, yet he doesn't do or say anything objectionable. The elaborate plot and contrived situation, while unusually detailed, are typical of the complexity that some dreams contain. Layered details compound excitement, and plot devices free dreamers from the slightest guilt or worry.

As mentioned, more typical vampire dreams of young adults are often far more edgy and dark than this one, focusing more on the neck-biting and the zombielike existence, with truly desperate attempts to escape. Some dream theorists have postulated that such images hint at struggles with addiction or feeling unable to make positive changes. Certainly the themes involved seem to hint at feelings of being overwhelmed, social pressure, attraction, and ambivalence.

It might seem likely that in the privacy of our own imaginations, we would not need quite so much elaboration, but sometimes even fantasies have many layers of permission-giving, and settings that create the illusion of danger with the guarantee of safety.

Starring in a Porno Movie

One woman has a favorite fantasy that she is an actress, starring in a porno movie. The movie producer is encouraging her to have real, rather than simulated sex, and she says she will decide when the time comes. The movie shows her as some kind of dominatrix dressed in leather and carrying a whip. She is visiting some men in a dungeon somewhere, who have not been in the company of a woman for some time. The men are naked, chained to walls, and some are staked out on the floor. She walks by the men and stares at them closely, and they each get an erection as she walks by. Many of them ejaculate just at the sight of her. She focuses on one man staked on the floor, who has an erection but has not yet ejaculated. She straddles him and decides at the last minute to have real sex.

There are a lot of plot devices here that make the fantasy safe and flexible. She gets to have the Goddess of Sex feeling, as those poor prisoners climax when she walks by. She is imagining being an actress who is pretending to have sex: that too is a lot of permission-giving. While she plays the role of a dominatrix, it is more about the wardrobe and accessories than about a set of behaviors. Also because of the layers of role-playing and dissociation involved in this fantasy, she gets to experience the physical sensations without identifying with the behaviors.

Conjugal Visits

While courting a real-life convict in prison seems like a dicey proposition, women do sometimes dream about paying conjugal visits to prisoners. This doesn't seem like an appealing dream date (why not the French Riviera instead)? These dreams are a good example of elaborate plots that move sexual action forward, and seem to heighten the heat by putting parameters around it.

In one dream the woman had been corresponding with a prisoner for a while. They decided to get together, and she began visiting him regularly. Something about him was impossible to resist, and she made arrangements to start paying him conjugal visits.

She was escorted into a small room where he was waiting for her. She was allowed to spend the night with him, and they had sex several times, unable to get enough of each other. The sex was vigorous, relentless. Whether it was the situation, the combination of their chemistry, or his understandably pent-up hunger, this was an extraordinarily erotic scene for her.

She described herself as not being the type of woman who would ever take an interest in prisoners or criminals. She is a young, hardworking, upwardly mobile type. So why was this dream so intoxicating and memorable, and why was this a prison scene rather than something more in line with her life-style?

This dream is another example of the elaborate plot devices that heighten erotic tone and remove the dreamer from her constraints and concerns. She is paired with someone who is extraordinarily virile, starved for sex, and who simulates danger, but is not really dangerous to her. The conjugal visit puts an enclosure around the scene, creating the expectation of sex, and nearly the requirement of sex. In many women's sex dreams the setting is quite important: If you are stuck in an elevator, snowed in at a mountain fire tower, or visiting a prison, the setting introduces sexuality, gives permission, and eliminates other distracting factors in one swoop.

So on one level this dream shows her being removed from her normal life, doing something exotic with simulated danger, and finding herself in a sexual capsule where there is nothing to do but sweat and have orgasms.

On an intrapsychic level it's very possible that many of us have parts of ourselves that have been exiled; the things we planned or loved before we got so busy get shelved or put on hold indefinitely. This could explain why the prisoner is so attractive, and why communing with him is so intoxicating. It's very possible to have a steamy sex dream that provides a good time, and to also discover that the lover in the dream reflects elements in your own personality or potentials.

This sounds bizarre, but as dreams are forming, feelings, memories, stored potentials seem to get tapped to flesh out characters and move the story along. This is why it can be worthwhile to reflect on the attributes of your dream lover, not only to see if you can learn something about what you prefer in a relationship or an encounter, but also to see if there is something you can learn about yourself and your life.

The Dapper Amputee

One woman dreamed that she was on a street corner waiting to cross the street, when an elegant gentleman caught her eye. She was instantly attracted to him and shocked by her feelings because his legs were amputated: He sat and propelled himself along on a small platform on wheels. On the other hand, he was very smartly dressed, with an old-fashioned elegance that was charming and attractive. She paused, and they struck up a brief conversation. She felt such a rush of recognition and love for him that she couldn't help but embrace him, and their lips met in a brief kiss. At the same time, however, she felt embarrassed and ashamed, hoping that no one would see her embracing this man. When she awoke, she sensed the dream might have special significance. The feeling of recognition and affection had rolled over her like a wave, and rocked her back in the dream. But the layers of mixed feelings were also a bit over-whelming. In the dream she didn't want anyone to see her be-having recklessly, nor did she want anyone to think she was "with" this man, whose appearance was so shocking. We had the opportunity to discuss this dream in our group, and the interpretation was intriguing. Often when a woman longs for something very specific to fulfill herself, she will dream of be-ing drawn to a lover who is forbidden, improper, or somehow "untouchable." The particular woman who had this dream is very compassionate and open-minded. If she fell in love with a disabled person in real life, she would not hesitate to follow her heart, nor would she care what other people thought of her choice. But in the dream she felt ashamed, almost guilty, and very afraid someone would see her with this astonishing man, who felt like her true love.

This woman is extremely successful in her professional field and has built a wonderful life for herself through diligence, a shrewd mind, and hard work. There is, however, a very poetic, introspective side to her, and she often toys with the idea of writing fiction. She particularly loves history and is something of a historical scholar. Like most people, she has heard that it is nearly impossible to break into publishing, and she is em-barrassed and circumspect about this particular fantasy. It is as if she does not want anyone to "catch" her longing to write, and does not want to expose this hunger, this love, to anyone's contempt or ridicule. She also feels at a disadvantage because writing seems to be one of those fields where, if you have not already done it, no one will help you get started. This may be why the handsome man was obviously wounded or damaged. Like an idea that "has no legs," he has probably been bumping along inside her heart for many years, patiently and graciously waiting for a time when his particular gifts might be given an outlet.

The gift of the dream was to reveal the starkness and the depth of her love for her untouchable talents. Her feelings rose like a ball of fire when she saw this man: passion, desire, affection, attraction, recognition, and fear all swamped her. All of us present in the group that night had a chance to examine how anticipatory scorn can prevent us from examining our passions in the light of day, and seeing what we can do to let them come to life. By looking into the complex mix of her own reactions in the dream, this woman has determined to follow the siren call of her impulse to write, wherever it may lead. She is not quitting her "day job" but is giving herself permission to embrace this side of herself.

Dream Key #23

Exploring Settings and Characters

Generally, the more elaborate and complex your dream, the more likely it is to contain symbolic elements that can tell you something valuable about your life. This doesn't mean that simple dreams are insignificant, it just means that when the mind goes to the ends of the earth to create a location, situation, or character, then there is usually a reason for that, and the reason has everything to do with *you*.

When you analyze or interpret a setting, its useful to define its characteristics and see if they tell you anything about what you like, what makes you feel sensual or free to enjoy yourself.

. . .

Here are some things to look for:

Privacy
Expectation of sex
Mitigating circumstances
Encapsulation
Lifted out of regular life
Variables that heighten eroticism
Unusual powers of seduction/attraction
Simulated danger/actual safety

Makes some notes about what the setting of your dream provides for you in terms of fantasy and freedom.

How might this translate into your love life? For example, so many of women's dreams take on intensity when they are set in encapsulated settings, where they are away from it all, where sex is expected, where they are freed from routine and normal responsibilities. This implies that getaways, vacation, and travel are not just clichés; we really do feel sexier when in a situation that is divergent from routine.

If your setting is unusual, does it imply anything symbolically about your current circumstances?

What about your dream lover? Is this person designed to fulfill a fantasy? If so, what qualities do you find sexy? Simulated danger-actual safety is big in dreams, and it's a hard one to find in real life. But other qualities, such as humor, fun, simpatico, and sense of adventure, are more easy to come by.

. . .

Describe the dream lover with a few adjectives. Do any of these adjectives apply to you? What steps might you take, safely and sanely, to move toward passion and connection in your life, not only romantically and physically, but even in the broadest sense?

CHAPTER TWENTY-FOUR

Updating Memories

A number of dreams involve a process that appears to be updating our memories. In these dreams, situations from the past appear and are altered to incorporate present conditions and loved ones. Typically we don't associate old relationships with post-traumatic stress syndrome, but our dreams appear to create healing scenes in some cases, as if they are involved in a process of delicately lifting scar tissue from our hearts.

The Healing Quilt

One woman had a serial recurring dream, that she lay upon her childhood bedspread and people would come to visit her there on the bed. In some cases the people were children, bringing toys and inviting her to play. In other dreams adolescent boys would come and kiss her, trying to get her interested in a little friendly sexual play. Often in these dreams she would reach an impasse and feel cold. Finally, in her thirties, she dreamed that a neighbor who had been a friend of the family came and sat on the bed, and apologized to her for molesting her as a child. In this final dream the man who had for so long loomed large in her memory seemed small. He also seemed milder, even harmless. After that the dreams of the old quilt disappeared, and she felt that in some manner this haunting memory had come full circle and been healed.

She had of course remembered her early experience, had come to terms with it, and was leading a full and happy life. This was not a dream that retrieved a suppressed incident. Instead her dreams seemed to assess the severity of this old wound over the years, and to mark her progress as it became a more distant memory. As she grew up, her life was rich and happy. The monster of the past became smaller and less powerful. When he visited her in her dream at the old scene of the crime, it was a peaceful meeting that marked a sense of official closure for her.

It is an interesting facet of trauma that sometimes we do not dream of the events themselves. Instead the dreaming mind may substitute something of similar magnitude or simply set new stories in a similar location, or bring a symbol from the past into new dreams.

The Bunk Bed

One woman who was cornered as an adolescent and molested in a high bunk bed has apparently no dreams dealing directly with the molestation itself. However, in her current relationships, when there is a problem with trust or she feels uncomfortable, she often dreams that she and her partner are in a bunk bed. To her unconscious mind, this is the place where trouble starts, and if this signal arises, she knows it is time to scrutinize the relationship and her feelings, because it is like a flare on the road for her.

Psychotherapists might suggest that her early trauma makes her prone to friction in her relationships. She would argue that undercurrents in the relationship are marked and brought forward by this special code in her dreams.

The Alternate Life

A less common theme has to do with dreams of alternative paths in life. These dreams let us explore the road not taken. What if you had married the person you turned down, instead of the one you chose? What if you had stayed in school and had not had children?

Many women report these dreams later in life, when there is really some distance to look back on. One woman reported that in her dream she had married her first sweetheart. They had lived and loved all these years together, and she had a vivid memory of *not* marrying her (real) husband. Every detail of this alternate life was complete and current, including their careers and family. She and her (dream) husband had some kind of argument, and to make amends, she bought him a leather jacket that he had been wanting. He worked nights and was asleep when she got home. She put it on the table next to the alarm clock on his side of the bed, so that it would be the first thing he saw when awoke. Then she went to sleep, hoping that this would help to mend fences.

When she awoke in the morning, her husband was still asleep, but the jacket was gone. She lay there puzzled and dismayed for a few seconds. Then the reality washed over her. The entire life she'd had had literally been a dream. She was looking over the shoulder of her real husband, and there was no leather jacket, just as there was no argument with a man she had not seen for twenty years. She lay in bed then and hugged herself with contentment. The dream the night before, while not *awful*, had certainly convinced her that she married the right man, had the right life, and was exactly where she was supposed to be.

Heart Surgery

One woman dreamed that she had to undergo heart surgery. When the surgeons opened her up, they found the problem: There was a foreign object in her heart. A sliver of granite was somehow lodged inside one of the arteries, and it was causing a blockage. In the dream she was awake during the surgery and could feel them taking the tiny little shard out of there.

This was the dream of a woman who had some bad memories of bitter times in the past. When she started a new and promising relationship, it was as if the dreaming mind did a bit of housecleaning. The heart surgery reflected a change going on in her emotions and implied that some healing was taking place. Granite is known for its hardness, obviously. The removal of this granite chip symbolically implies that something hard in her was being released, and that, with time, whatever felt "blocked" in her feelings would be softened and reconnected.

Dreams of heart surgery are fairly common, especially among women. Although in some cases they may be associated with actual medical conditions, in cases where that makes no sense, it can be useful to consider whether some kind of emotional healing or change is taking place. Symbolically, the heart is more than just the romantic seat of Hallmark messages; it is the center, the core, of the emotional matrix so to speak. When we undergo a fundamental emotional change in our lives, it may be marked by dreams involving the heart.

No More Scars

Just as the heart can be a powerful emblem of emotion, so scars can appear in dreams that deal with emotional and psychological wounding. In these types of dreams women take care to conceal their scars, either by clothing, bandages, or by staying in enclosed areas.

One woman dreamed that she wanted to leave the hospital-like setting where she lived because there was a young man she was interested in. Like a damsel in a fairy tale, she longed to be with him, but stayed inside because she was so scarred. At some point, though, the nurses came to her and showed her in a mirror that her scars had long since healed. She ran her hands over her skin in disbelief; it was smooth. How long had she wasted staying inside, when there was nothing wrong with her anymore? She was healed.

This woman was very active and not at all a fragile, retiring sort. Yet evidently there was some aspect of her that she had tucked away, and kept protected because it had been so horribly hurt that it seemed better to keep this energy permanently sheltered.

The dream is a kind of coming-out signal, dramatically informing her that her scars have healed, there is nothing wrong with her, and there is no further need to keep this energy out of the world.

The Tattooed Lady

Tattoos figure frequently in the dreams of women, particularly women who are changing or acquiring some kind of independence. In these dreams the women get outlandish tattoos, and far from regretting their impulsivity or the process, they lounge around admiring their incredibly sensual appearance.

One woman who went through a gritty divorce dreamed of getting a particularly sexy tattoo across her back and another on one cheek of her bottom. In the dream she found the tattoos glorious. They made her feel differently about her body, as if she were a siren; dangerous and sensual. In the dream she tested her theory with a new lover, who helped christen her tattoos and seemed very appreciative of the artwork and of her.

She found this dream so provocative, that she later went out and got a tattoo, as much like the dream one as she could. I had a chance to inquire later whether she was experiencing the sorts of things she had hoped for, and she replied cryptically, "So far, so good."

Catching the Serial Killer

It's hard for some people to settle down. Some say that the longer you're single, the more accustomed you are to being on your own. Maybe it's true that we get set in our ways. Some women have told me that they suspect they have a kind of mechanism in their psyches that keeps them single. They like their partners, but it's like they have their finger on the button of an ejection seat all the time. They can almost feel themselves waiting for a reason to push the button.

One woman had a dream that helped her get a handle on this "mechanism" and to operate more consciously in her relationships. Since she eventually married and seems happy, maybe it worked.

In her dream there was a serial killer on the loose. This was someone who had been around for ten years or so, systematically killing people every six months to a year. The police were not able to track him very well. He would commit a murder and then just disappear. There weren't any signs of him really, and no one knew where he went underground between the killings. The dreamer sometimes felt his presence outside, but when she looked often she couldn't be sure if she saw a shadow move outside on the street below. One night, she had her boyfriend over and they were messing around in the living room. She happened to see something move outside and looked down and could see a figure dart into a darkened doorway. She froze and knew it was the killer. Then she remembered there had been some theory that the killer was attracted to young lovers; she had forgotten that until just now.

In the tradition of amateur sleuths everywhere, she pulled out a notebook and began writing down what she knew about the killer. She and her boyfriend decided they would try to catch him by using themselves as decoys and trying to flush him out. They would involve the police in their plan and see if, together, they could catch this guy.

A period of dark, suspenseful watching ensues, as the dreamer records clues and poses in front of the window in her lover's arms to see if she can draw out the killer of young lovers.

The dream did not provide her with a happy ending. Before she had come to a sense of what it was about, the whole thing seemed creepy, scary, and harebrained. She looked back on her dream-bravado with incredulity. In the language of dreams, death sometimes simply means "endings" or "change." This serial killer may in fact have symbolized her tendency to snuff out relationships as they wore thin or disappointed her. The ability to make hard choices and get out of something that's bad for you is a good thing. Yet she did have the sense that leaving was her best and favorite problem-solving strategy. Since she had been dating and having relationships about ten years, the history of this serial killer seemed to coincide with her love life.

What seems important about this dream is not that we have little exit-agents in our personalities that help us leave. More pivotal is the fact that the dream showed the shadow side of this mechanism. The serial killer is a destroyer, a saboteur who skulks around in the darkness plotting destruction. The dreamer herself is on the side of life, and it is the proximity of her relationship that seems to draw out the murderous aspect. This dream not only gives a rough sketch of the patterns, but it also represents the first time the dreamer becomes aware of the pattern. In her lover's arms, she spots the killer darting for cover. Not only does she glimpse what is going on, but she decides that together, she and her boyfriend will "catch the killer." She will keep track of the clues and involve the police. In real life, like many women, she used journaling to try and sort out her different feelings and experiences. Perhaps the "listing of clues" was a reference to this practice. Involving the police seems like a metaphor for paying attention, staying lucid, and exerting power.

As it happened, I believe the boyfriend of that time period did fall prey to the killer, as it were. But the dreamer did find and fall in love with another man, with no sign of casualties in sight. They have been together for some years, so evidently the killer, along the way, was caught.

Dream Key #24

Updating Files

You don't have to wait for your dreams to spontaneously update your history. You can work with your dreams consciously and help to realize how far you've come and what is within your power. Finish the sentences below without thinking too much first, and notice what comes out. Write your statements in your journal.

1. I no longer have to worry about . . .

2. I never thought it would happen, but I finally . . .

3. Something I've recently learned about myself is . . .

4. One thing I've always wanted and have achieved is . . .

5. Something I have let go of is . . .

6. One change I deliberately made was to . . .

CHAPTER TWENTY-FIVE

Erotic Passages

There is little doubt that we have different preoccupations and priorities at different times of life. Knowing when you're moving through a "passage" can be helpful because it normalizes things and can let you know what to expect. Our dreams in general tend to have many different focuses as we move through life. Our erotic dreams and fantasies change through time as well.

Crushing Success

In early teen years, dreams often focus like a tracking device on the location of a "crush" and the odds of romantic feelings being reciprocated. Girls dream prolifically about their current crush being thrown together with them by fate, and in a private moment, with time and the outside world suspended, they learn that he shares their feelings. The situations and plot mechanisms change, as does the crush. The elements of the dreams that seem fairly consistent are the opportunity to be alone, the disclosure of affection, and the privacy. These are not dreams of having sex in the back row of the bleachers, or being invited to be an extra on a music video. These are private, almost sacred moments, not about admiration or flaunting, but about genuinely being liked.

One young woman dreamed of being at a school function that involved staying after school and helping with the production of a group project. She went outside and took a break. While returning, she encountered her crush, and they took time to sit together in room that wasn't being used. They sat talking quietly, and she waited to hear if he might say something more personal. In a rush he began to tell her that he had liked her for a long time, but had been embarrassed to approach her. He took her hand, and they kissed.

In real life apparently things had not yet developed between them, and this girl, like many of us, wondered if perhaps the dream held out the promise that things might yet unfold. As a predictor of future connections, these dream perhaps are not suitable devices of divination. But they do help young women fulfill the fantasy of hearing the specific words from the specific person they care about. They also help them have a virtual rehearsal of the next phase in their social schedule. If this crush doesn't come through, one of the crushes yet to come will.

While some teens may be having much more raunchy erotic dreams, these crush scenes are touchingly innocent and genuine. They are not so much erotic as romantic, the point of the exercise is affection and recognition; being liked back. In later years we may have other agendas as well, but in a very real sense this is always what we are up to: loving and hoping to be loved.

One notable quality to these dreams is a kind of worshipful purity of projection. There isn't anything here about what the girl wants or needs or expects. She is not a being full of feelings hoping for a partner who will fit. She is like a flower turning toward the sun. In this story everything she feels seems inspired because of the quality of the crush. It is no wonder that so much appears to hinge on his response. By implication, if things don't go well, or he goes away, all those potential feelings go with him.

Fantasies during this time, and of this genre, are almost identical to the dreams. Being alone with the crush is a miracle of circumstance that is coveted in these fantasies. For some reason, privacy equals intimacy, and these fantasies involve the opportunity to be alone. The crush then says everything she has been wanting to hear. In these fantasies further sexual exploration often occurs, but typically these are not yet erotic scenes. The intensity focuses most upon the declarations of affection and the return of feelings.

The Vampire-Slayer Years

After the simplicity of the crush fantasies, young women seem to go wild in their dreams. These themes are focused on sexual power and the validation of desirability. They are no longer quivering and vulnerable, hoping to be liked. Something supercharges them into young sirens bringing men to their knees through ultra-desirability.

These dreams sometimes involve a theme of exhibitionism, like the Vampire Initiation Party in an earlier chapter. These dreams contain considerably more sexual action and eroticism, but it is often pointed toward proof of power and sexuality, rather than directly at sensual pleasure.

One woman had a dream that she was leaning against a young man's car, wearing a tight strapless sundress. She could feel him looking at her breasts and could feel her nipples were visible in the fabric. She leaned back on the warm panel of his car and rubbed her backside slowly back and forth as if she were polishing the car. "You," he growled at her, his erection now visibly growing in his pants. "You're driving me crazy." She laughed at him and he sprang forward, pulling down the top of her sundress, cupping her breasts and kissing her. He pushed her back against car and pressed his erection into her crotch.

This scene has several elements of this genre of eroticism. In these dreams women tend to wear and revel in provocative outfits. The dreamer also delights in giving the young man a hard-on. She is causing him some trouble and that is, after all the point of the scene. She controls the action by being enticing and mischievous. She moves her body, his body responds, and he lets her know she is indeed something he can't resist.

Finally the dream also suggests that this woman is not about to play second fiddle to a guy's car. She stands between him and his car leaning on his pride and joy. He doesn't leap over to get her away from the car's finish; he leaps over to pull down her top with shaking hands and grind his erection into her. She is the most important thing, the victor.

Clinching the Deal

Fantasies during this phase involve the consummation of relationship through seductive power so great it that ensures the future. These fantasies blend eroticism with sexual leverage. For this to be satisfying there usually needs to be some exhibitionism or public admiration as well.

One young woman repeatedly fantasized that a man she admired would come by her apartment building while she was out sunning herself. She would look up as a shadow crossed her and find him staring at her. Without saying anything to anyone, he would lie down on top of her, in front of everyone, and kiss her passionately as he explored her body and pressed himself into her. Although not explicitly detailed or rehearsed in the fantasy, this would be the beginning of their passionate and long-lasting relationship. Likely part of what made this fantasy satisfying was the presence of onlookers, witnesses to her power and his compulsion to have her.

These fantasies are essentially an all-in-one delightful daydream. You are proven to be so seductive that the person you want is overwhelmed and has to have you. You get the attention, sex, and pleasure with the person of your choice, and you have also somehow mysteriously clinched the deal, by virtue of supreme desirability. He's yours now, not just for a moment of intoxicating dry humping, but forever. It's pretty satisfactory.

I've Come for You

Somewhere after the phase of being proven a hot property, women begin to dream and fantasize about being recognized as unique. Not unique because of attractiveness alone, but unique because of you. That doesn't mean the sexy stuff goes away, or is discounted, but there is much more to the plan now. In these dreams, one of the intoxicating moments is actually eye contact.

One woman dreamed of meeting a man while walking along a beach. They talked and felt some common stirring. They held hands and clambered upward to find a private place back from the shoreline. Moving toward some trees, they held hands and looked into each other's eyes. When they found a quiet place, partially sheltered by trees, they sat down together, and he slipped her blouse away from her shoulder. They kissed and lay down, feeling each other's warmth.

In this dream the woman is having a little fantasy about a chance encounter that is pregnant with deeper meaning. These two are connecting. They aren't just stirring because they want to have sex, although that is what moves the action along. But the reason they have to run off and do it right now is because they *know* each other. He "gets it" somehow that she is this special person of unique depth, and she gets it that he senses this about her. This is really what the heat is about. He isn't complimenting her figure, and she isn't wearing anything special or memorable that is part of the story. She remembered looking into his eyes, and that they felt each other's warmth. No one sees that she has moved him; we are back to a theme of privacy again. Like the early fantasy of the crush, this kind of sharing is private and special, not about feeling sexy because others know you are having fun.

There is a hint of destiny to this scene. Often these dreams feel as if the right person has shown up at the right time. He has come for you. Not to rescue you or to prove you are hot. He has come because he can see who you are.

Dreams of recognition and intimacy tend to predominate as wish-fulfillment themes for some time for women, and indeed can appear at any stage of the life span after they initially appear.

Aphrodite's Beeper

After a while the chaos factor of adult life takes its toll and intrudes in our dreams. As we marry, have families, ramp up careers, and age, our erotic dreams expand to cover more territory. While some explore rich fantasy, others reflect the factors that impinge on our opportunities and energy for sex. These dreamers are old enough to know what they find sexy in partners, in situations, and in themselves. They are often so busy and responsible for so many things and people that their erotic dreams are peppered with interruptions and flukes that short-circuit satisfaction.

One woman dreamed that she gave a coworker a ride home, and when they reached his house they sat in the car and talked. They had a strong attraction, and they were both finding excuses to keep the conversation going so that he wouldn't feel he had to go in. She was feeling increasingly hot, physically and sexually. She kept wriggling around in the seat because, on top of everything else, her panties seemed to have ridden up and were stimulating her. She needed to just lift up her hips, reach down, and adjust things, but she didn't want to be conspicuous, so she just ground her hips around hoping for some improvement. Her friend, of course, recognized the writhing of a woman in a bad way when he saw it, and he swiftly moved over to her. They kissed for a blissfully sweet moment. And then her beeper went off.

She awoke to find her alarm was going off. Although we all have alarm clocks, this dream is typical of the happy erotic scene just starting to show promise that gets nipped in the bud by some interruption. Our beepers, cell phones, and so on are images of the modern life that "owns" us in a sense. Even our fantasies are not sacred, and we can't seem to hide from the things that pull our strings.

Old Faithful

One woman had an intriguing dream that she was trying to find time alone before her kids and husband got home. She wanted to lie down, masturbate, relax, and take a nice nap. She stole away and got settled, got out her vibrator, got situated, and found the batteries were dead. She threw it back in the drawer, thinking, "So much for Old Faithful."

This vignette is an echo of the greater theme of these dreams. When, miraculously, circumstances do give her some time for rest and self-stimulation, her batteries have gone dead!

Women are in a tough game of balancing energy, opportunity, and time. Yet with all these factors pressing in, our fantasies and erotic themes do become more exotic and provocative throughout the life span.

Dancing on the Ceiling

One woman dreamed that as she slept she was drawn upward out of her body and was floating in the air above the bed. She felt something like a magnetic power was holding her there suspended. Far from being an alarming sensation, this was a fluttery sensual feeling, like a wind caressing her, holding her in the air. Then she sensed she was not alone and felt someone pressing behind her.

A pair of arms encircled her and whoever it was began nuzzling her neck. The combination of the floating and the warmth and the caresses were wonderful. She was content, but asked him who he was. He seemed embarrassed. "I'm just someone you used to know," he said. Then she realized who it was, a man from her distant past who had been a favorite lover, and a warm memory. She turned then to face him, and they swirled around in the air together, dancing in space. At one point as they held each other, they were perfectly upside down, dancing on the ceiling.

This gentle dream has elements of spirituality, since she lifts out of her body and floats carefree in air. Also she is reunited with an old love. They gently revolve and dance, defying all laws, savoring each other's company and the magic of the moment. The sexuality is implied in everything in the dream; the very air is like a warm breeze caressing her skin. This is not a dream with anything to prove; it is like a gift, lifting the dreamer out of time, out of her body. It seems important that gravity is suspended and that she is reunited with her old lover in this floating dance. It is romantic, spectral. The sensuality is liberated from the physical context, and we see that it exists beyond the boundaries that normally seem to confine it. We hope that we are more than our bodies. This dream suggests that perhaps sexuality, passion, and eroticism are more than what we know as well.

Dream Key #25

Themes and Passages

Knowing what gives you pleasure and what you value at any given time can help you to maximize the odds of getting what you want, and minimize the odds of calamity. Review the statements below and see which apply to you most.

I fantasize about people I know and care about.

In my fantasies the other person tells me how he feels; I want to hear it.

I consider how I look and what I am wearing in a fantasy; that is part of it.

I like to think of meeting someone who will understand me, who "gets" it.

I fantasize about feeling I'm on track, with privacy and space to savor someone.

I fantasize about unusual situations and whole-body relaxation as well as sex.

I fantasize about getting some sleep.

I fantasize about being able to take time, and have time taken with me.

I fantasize about meeting someone who will fit my world and my interests.

My favorite dreams are those of having uncomplicated fun sex.

My favorite dreams are those of feeling connected and understood.

My favorite dreams have vivid sensual feelings and clear detail.

Conclusion

The exploration of our dreams usually begins out of curiosity, but the additional benefits of that exploration are without limit. The content of your dreams, the meaning you derive, and the benefits you will enjoy from understanding them is a treasure you already own. If you have enjoyed this look into your own dreaming mind, then make it a point to talk with others who may want to explore dreams on a regular basis. The process lends itself to group sharing, and it doesn't matter how much or how little experience anyone in the group may have. Listening respectfully and staying open-minded are really all it takes to begin to unravel these mysteries and to claim the prize they often hold, both for the dreamer, and for those who help to explore the dream.

You may want to start a monthly or biweekly dream group in your home, having friends bring written copies of dreams to share. If you want to take a class or join an existing dream sharing group, look at local bookstore bulletin boards, alternative press publications, and community college classes. These groups are often quiet and private, and often there is little or no fee involved.

If you prefer to work alone, just keep up your journal and

select some way of highlighting the dreams that feel important. Over time, even as little as a few months, you will begin to have a real handle on your unique dreaming style, and you'll see how your intuitive dreams are commenting on your relationships and your deepest passions. The richness of your emotional nature and the wisdom of your mind and spirit are woven through your dreams each night. Make it your intention to embrace them and see where they take you.

Appendix One

Shortcut to Erotic Dreams

If you're interested in having more erotic dreams, here are a few suggestions.

1. As circumstances allow, read something sexy right before bed. Alternatively, watch a sexy video shortly before bed.

2. Masturbate slightly, but not enough to have an orgasm. Then go to sleep.

3. Do some stretches and yoga postures before going to sleep. Lie on your back and lift up your hips, or rock your hips side to side as if to stretch the lower back.

4. Wear something to bed in which you feel attractive, whether anyone is there or not.

5. Consciously think as you go to sleep that you would like an erotic dream. Then just relax.

6. Keep something beside the bed so that if you do have an intriguing dream, you can write it down or tape-record it.

7. If you have a lover, ask that person to share their erotic dreams with you.

8. Ask friends appropriately if they have had any interesting sex dreams they can remember.

9. If you notice yourself having disrupted erotic dreams frequently, ask you unconscious mind to give you sexy dreams without ruining them. Ask if there is some other way you could get the "message," if there is one. This seems to work with taking the terror out of nightmares, so it stands to reason it may take the interruptions out of sexual dreams, too.

APPENDIX TWO

Sexual Symbolism

Understanding the meaning of a dream symbol requires evaluating three things.

1. Context. The context of the dream or scene in which the image appeared is important. Only you know if the dream was scary or fun-loving. King Kong could be a monster or a goofy friend, depending upon the dream's tone and your associations to a particular image. If you refer to the ideas about symbolic meaning here, or in any guide, keep in mind that the genre or type of dream you had is also a key factor in deciding the meaning of a symbol. No symbol is necessarily good or bad; evaluate it in terms of the scene in which it appeared.

2. Personal associations. Your personal associations to a symbol or a character are likely to be unique. If you aren't sure what you think of a particular symbol, describe it in one sentence as if you were defining it for a very simple dictionary. Is Batman a creepy mutant, or is he a misunderstood hero who is never properly thanked? Your personal interpretation of a person or an object is the thing that matters most when translating a symbol into whatever it really represents.

3. **Typical interpretations.** Sometimes it is truly hard to get a personal definition or to know where to start with a baffling image. In such cases, one way to get started decoding a dream is to refer to broad ideas of modern symbolism, and what many people have already observed from Dreamwork. These are not rules that will necessarily hold true for everyone, but when you are stuck or have no idea why a weird gizmo appeared in your dream, these general interpretations can get you started. If you feel the general interpretation is somehow not right for you, then trust that instinct and move from the general interpretation to what you believe fits for you. Sometimes we don't know what we believe or what is inside us until someone offers the "wrong" advice, and then suddenly our personal truth comes into clear focus. Every symbol has a positive and a negative potential, which can only be tracked by the dreamer herself.

For example, driving downhill could represent freedom, being "over the hump," and feeling a task is all downhill from here. In another context, driving downhill could mean racing out of control in a downward spiral. Only you know how the dream *felt* at the time, and your sense of the positive or negative qualities is the ultimate detective service in solving the mysteries of your dreams.

The descriptions below should merely serve as a reference to get you started thinking symbolically and should be fleshed out or countered with your own feelings and memory of the dream.

AFFAIRS When affairs are referenced, this may represent connections being forged, either with a quality or a person. When there is guilt involved, this hints that there are complicated issues involved.

AMPUTATION Amputation symbolizes the feeling of loss of a part of yourself, or any dramatic change that leaves you feeling vulnerable.

APPLAUSE Applause typically represents pubic recognition, or the dreamer's sense that it is acceptable to "go public" with something.

APPLES Perhaps due to the biblical reference of Adam and Eve, apples often appear in dreams that are sorting through a specific relationship or the complexity of relationships. An apple core may reference the "core" of an issue.

AQUARIUM These represent a special environment necessary for the health and happiness of living creatures with unique needs. Damaged, neglected aquariums suggest emotional starvation of some kind.

BABY Babies typically symbolize new projects and potentials. Often the baby's age in the dream can provide a clue as to what is being represented; the "new thing" in your life will be the same age as the child.

BAKING Baking symbolizes the creative process, like a form of incubation or "cooking" up an idea. Baking can also represent pregnancy.

BARBARIANS Nameless barbarian groups that threaten homes and villages in dreams can represent threatening influences in real life. The threat can be from a group, or from the harsh side of a loved one who sometimes exhibits "attack" energy.

BAREFOOT Being barefoot hints at a sense of vulnerability and sometimes uncertainty about being prepared or having a definite role in a particular setting.

BEACHES Beaches often symbolize a place of transition in the dreamer's life, particularly when the familiar is over and the new chapter is still relatively unknown.

BEAR Bears often represent threatening male energy, particularly if they are savage or scary. Recurring bear-chase dreams may reference an old, hurtful experience from the dreamer's past.

BEDROOM This may reflect the part of your life that deals with sexuality, intimacy, and privacy.

BIRTH Births represent the beginning of a situation, relationship, or phase of your life. Naturally if you are pregnant, the birth can be a rehearsal of the birth process ahead, often filled with peculiar challenges that are not predictive but may process anxiety.

BOATS The relationship depicted as a vessel. The shape it's in, and the control you have over navigation are sometimes symbolic of how you're feeling in the relationship.

BROKEN GLASS Broken promises, shattered expectations, hurt feelings. It may also signify a situation that is emerging into a crisis.

BUFFALO A white buffalo may represent something sacred to the dreamer. More typically a herd of thundering buffalo may symbolize feeling stampeded or "buffaloed" by something or someone.

BUILDINGS Buildings tend to symbolize the activity or function they stand for in the dream. Factories represent productivity, prisons confinement, churches religion, and so on.

CABIN A cabin often represents the private life of a couple or person. This is the space in which you are together, without judgment or the opinions of the outside world.

CAKE Cake seems to reflect a current situation or a style of relating. Do you just want the frosting and throw the rest away? Or do you find that after you've eaten the cake, it cost $20 per slice? Do you serve it up to everyone else so that there is none left for you?

CANDY Sweet food can symbolize sweet experiences or loving kindness. Dreams of trying to get some candy may reflect a hunger for emotional sweetness or nurturance.

CARESS A caress is typically a positive reference to feeling accepted and loved. When unwanted, it symbolizes emotional trespass of some kind.

CARS Your own car (even when it is fictional) represents your self and your identity. A shared car tends to represent a relationship or social body. A threatening vehicle often symbolizes a person who "runs you over" or pushes you around.

CATS Cats are associated with feminine energy, that is, the feminine side of you, or of another person. They may even reflect gynecological health or illness.

CAVES Caves may represent shelter from the storms of life; they may also represent the womb or a return to feminine nurturance.

CONDOMS Protection, against the "dangers" of intimacy, either emotional or physical, and the intention to make a connection.

CRABS Crabs typically refer to "being crabby" or cranky. They may also refer to cancer, or a "cancerous" situation, or to traveling sideways, or even to the negative cost of impulsive contacts, such as genital crabs.

CRAZINESS When someone is insane in a dream, it may reflect unpredictability or impaired judgment in waking life, either with respect to a specific situation, or more globally.

CRUISE SHIPS Typically these ships reflect the state of your relationship, whether it is "smooth sailing" or encountering "troubled waters."

CURTAINS Curtains represent veiled situations that are

still unclear; when there is more to the story than meets the eye.

DANCING Dancing often symbolizes sex; although it may more generally represent freedom of expression.

DARTS Darts typically represent critical comments, quick attacks, or put-downs, where retaliation or defense is all but impossible.

DINOSAURS Dinosaurs tend to represent scary things from the past that are poorly understood, but rear up from time to time.

DOGS Dogs may represent men, male energy, or loyalty.

DUNGEONS Like all places of imprisonment, dungeons tend to symbolize situations in life that box us in; or our own tendency to cast a side of ourselves into exile.

EARRINGS Earrings may symbolize the opinions we hear or the "tape recordings" we mentally play for ourselves.

EARS Ears represent what we hear, and the mental atmosphere around us.

E-MAIL E-mail can represent the mental conversation between you and another.

FIRE While fire can represent passion and chemistry, it is often associated with anger and explosive situations. Dreams of being caught in fires should be taken seriously as potential cautionary dreams.

FISH Fish in an aquarium typically represent the dreamer's emotional nature. Fish in bed, especially small ones, may represent sperm.

FOREIGN OBJECTS When a foreign object is found in part of the body, this suggests that a belief or teaching from someone else has "gotten under your skin" and is impacting your intimate life.

FROGS Potential partners. In cases where the frog is a magical creature, it may represent intuition.

FUNGUS Negative growth or an opportunistic element in a situation or relationship.

GENITALS Genitalia represent masculine or feminine sexuality, power, and intimacy. Extra genitals in a dream are not a bad thing; they suggest integration of power and potentials.

GESTATION The time when something new is definitely on the way but has not yet arrived.

GIANTS Oversized people (or things) tend to represent situations that loom large from our perspective; something considered "a big deal."

HORSES Horses often represent the vital and sexual side of the dreamer. They may also symbolize physical health and emotional freedom.

HOUSES Dream houses often symbolize the psychic space you're currently in. The conditions of the home may match your subjective reality.

ICEBERG Something potentially problematic, usually to a relationship; look for "hard feelings" or "frozen emotions." Expect that there may be much more there than what is initially visible.

IGNITION SWITCH The part of you that turns on, or gets things started.

INCEST Incest usually represents a violation of boundaries. It may symbolize psychological enmeshment, as in working for friends. Finally, some incest simply registers the similarity between a current love interest and a family member.

INFIDELITY Infidelity usually represents emotional betrayal or some kind of disappointed expectation.

KANGAROO An exotic, bewildering situation or behavior.

KNIFE Knives can represent criticism, "cutting remarks." However, they often symbolize unwanted sexual attention, as in being pursued or stalked.

LADDER Ladders often represent situations that must be

handled in a step-by-step manner. They can also refer to progress in life, such as a professional ladder, or spiritual evolution.

LEAVES Often leaves are a pun on "leaving" a person, situation, or place.

LEFT The left side is associated with the feminine, intuitive, creative, and flowing nature of life. The left side may also pertain specifically to mother, or to a particular woman.

LINES Lines typically symbolize rules, guidelines, and expectations. Whether in a coloring book, on a highway, or your pants-leg, lines are connected with logical consistency.

MARRIAGE When it is obviously symbolic, a dream marriage represents the unification of energies or potentials that have previously been separate.

MICE Mice typically represent details and minor worries that seem to multiply and overtake the big picture.

MIRRORS Mirrors often symbolize the self-concept or the way you feel others see you.

MOON The moon is associated with feminine energy, introversion, and subtle insights such as intuition.

NAILS Nails may present a pun on "getting nailed" sexually. They may also reflect an aggressive, dominating energy that may be controlling or restrictive.

NARCOTICS Drugs usually pertain to a sense of intoxication, and in the extreme, the potential for addiction and destructive tendencies.

NEWBORN A newborn symbolizes a new situation or opportunity that needs shelter and nurturance before it can flourish and grow.

NIGHTTIME Dreams set at night hint that the situation under scrutiny has elements of the unknown and the mysterious. When we cannot "see" well visually in a dream, this implies that we are having trouble with perception in some way in real life.

OFFICIALS Officials often symbolize the external values or expectations in a given situation. These are the "rules" in life, and they often appear to inhibit our freedom. Sometimes these rules are external; often they reflect our own fears about getting what we want.

OPERATIONS Surgeries tend to represent changes, either planned or unexpected. Symbolically surgeries reflect a reorganization or change in perspective.

OPPOSITION The forces in a situation, or in your psyche, that run counter to your stated objective or agenda.

PACKAGES Packages symbolize situations or potentials that sometimes take the stage in life. Often this is "the thing" that you must address next in order to have what you want or solve a problem.

PACKING The act of preparing for something that is important to you.

PENIS Typically a penis is associated with masculine power and potentials.

PIE Pies often symbolize the self, the whole. They may also represent the resources or energy available to a group.

PLANES In sexual dreams, planes can either represent the transcendent ride of passion, or may represent an erect phallus.

QUIZZES Quizzes and exams often represent hurdles that are currently impacting progress. Usually the dreamer is quite earnest about expectations and places more pressure on herself than anyone else.

RABID ANIMALS Rabid animals may represent hidden rage or unpredictable patterns in someone close. Just as these animals should be considered dangerous, so the real-life situation should be dealt with cautiously.

RAFTS Rafts represent makeshift mechanisms for surviving change, transition, or rough times.

RAILROAD Railroad tracks and trains often symbolize logical, linear, conventional thinking. Any "ride" can symbolize sex: When this is the case, the ride is usually fun, rather than frightening or claustrophobic.

RAPE Rape can represent any kind of violation that takes away choice, is highly troubling, and feels very personal.

RAZORS Razors represent sharp words or the potential for someone to lash out.

RESTAURANTS Eating establishments typically symbolize opportunities to choose what kind of experience you intend to have. If the menu is limited, or everybody gets to choose but you, consider whether you are feeling boxed-in, or left out, in a current situation.

RINGS Rings often represent promises and loyalty. Rings from a beloved can hint at the quality of the promises being made, rings from family or from oneself hint at long-standing promises about your walk through life.

ROWBOATS Sometimes rowboats symbolize the "work" involved in a relationship. This is particularly true if the dream deals with the oars and who is doing the rowing.

SADISM Sadistic punishment in dreams usually reflects a "punitive" streak in a relationship where blame is an ongoing part of the unspoken arrangement.

SNAKES Snakes most frequently represent trouble, especially when there are several at once. However, a single snake may be a phallic symbol, particularly if it appears in the bedroom.

SPIDERS When they appear in the bedroom, or another

intimate setting, spiders can represent the negative side of sexuality and relationship—the "dark" side—that can be scary and hurtful.

STARS   Stars sometimes symbolize destiny or special timing.

STORMS   Weather often reflects the current emotional climate of the dreamer's situation. Stormy weather is a metaphor for turbulent emotions.

SUNSHINE   Dreams set in sunny surroundings typically reflect positive feelings and good times.

TATTOOS   Tattoos in dreams typically deal with taking back one's power, almost in the shamanic sense of "soul" retrieval. For example, becoming sexy after a divorce, becoming powerful after being discounted or devalued.

TEETH   Teeth represent the sort of "grain" of your personality. When a situation, person or relationship goes against the grain, there is erosion, and teeth-loss dreams may occur.

TRAINS   Like railroad tracks, trains tend to represent something that goes in a straight line, like a train of thought or a situation that, once started, is difficult to alter or stop.

TREES   Individual trees can represent new growth and progress, as well as the potential for life to flourish in the future.

UMBILICUS   Dreams about the umbilical area often deal

with issues pertaining to one's relationship with Mom, and how that pertains to current relationships and identity.

UTERUS The uterus can represent actual childbearing ability and sexual feelings, but it is more often symbolic of the ability to carry an idea or plan through to fruition.

VAGINA Feminine and sexual energy.

VULTURES Any person or situation that intervenes after the "end" of something or makes it's living by showing up after a "death" of some kind.

WALLS Separations between people, situations, or aspects of the self.

WATER Emotion, fluidity, uncharted regions of the psyche. In showers and bathes water represents restoration and nurturance.

WHALES The original self, undamaged, full of peace and power.

ZOMBIES Zombies represent robotic living, or automatic behaviors.

Suggested Resources

1. *Finding Your Perfect Match: 8 Ways to Find Lasting Love Through True Compatibility*, by Pepper Schwartz, PhD.

   This book gives great ideas about real compatibility, and why it is definitely the place to start, if you're serious about your happiness.

2. *Our Dreaming Mind*, by Robert Van De Castle, PhD.

   This is *the* book on contemporary research in dream studies and gives a great overview of the now-exploding field.

3. *Women's Bodies, Women's Dreams*, by Patricia Garfield, PhD.

   This wonderful book explores all sorts of dreams women have that relate to their bodies, health, aging, and emotions.

4. The International Association for the Study of Dreams. Website: www.asdreams.org.

The association is a nonprofit group from all over the world comprising scientists, teachers, therapists, artists, and people who have discovered the profundity and magic of their dreams. If you're getting hooked on dreams, you'll want to visit their website and see the research being done. They may have a conference in your area, so be sure to look for meetings, classes, and regional conferences.

INDEX